THE CAVEMAN'S
PREGNANCY COMPANION

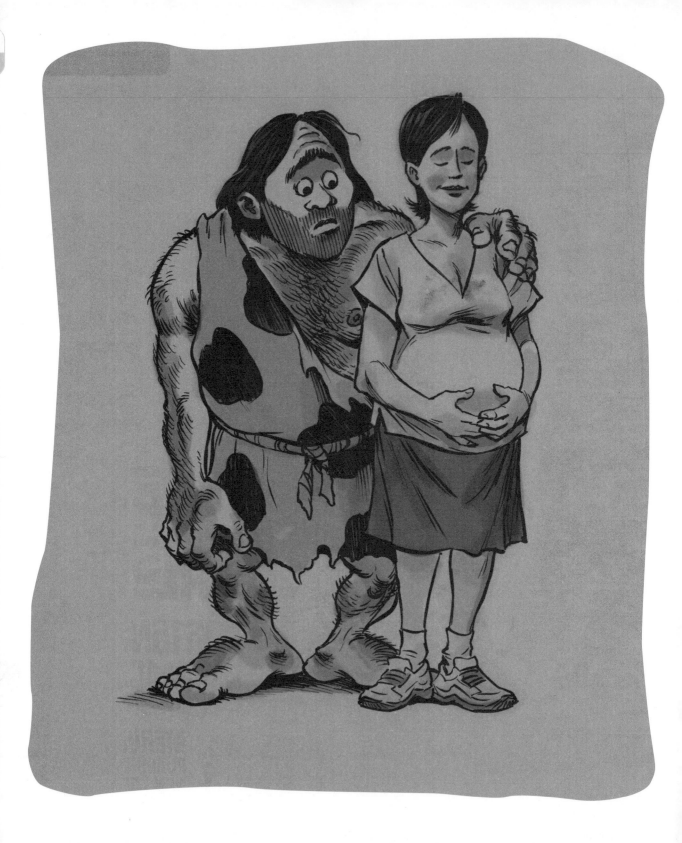

THE CAVEMAN'S PREGNANCY COMPANION

A SURVIVAL GUIDE FOR EXPECTANT FATHERS

DAVID PORT AND JOHN RALSTON

BRIAN M. RALSTON, M.D., FELLOW, AMERICAN ACADEMY OF FAMILY PHYSICIANS · CONSULTANT

GIDEON KENDALL, ILLUSTRATOR

STERLING PUBLISHING NEW YORK

We cavemen would be lost in the modern world
without rock-solid women to inspire and guide us.
This book is dedicated to our wives, Diana and
Emily, our daughters, Juliette, Jane, and Lila, our
mothers, Bridget and Candace, and our grandmothers,
Miriam, Ellen, Florence, and Jacqueline.

PUBLISHED BY STERLING PUBLISHING CO., INC.
387 PARK AVENUE SOUTH, NEW YORK, NY 10016

PREPARED BY
SCOTT & NIX, INC.
150 WEST 28TH STREET
SUITE 1103
NEW YORK, NY 10001-6103
WWW.SCOTTANDNIX.COM

DISTRIBUTED IN CANADA BY STERLING PUBLISHING
C/O CANADIAN MANDA GROUP, 165 DUFFERIN STREET
TORONTO, ONTARIO, CANADA M6K 3H6

DISTRIBUTED IN THE UNITED KINGDOM
BY GMC DISTRIBUTION SERVICES
CASTLE PLACE, 166 HIGH STREET, LEWES
EAST SUSSEX, ENGLAND BN7 1XU

DISTRIBUTED IN AUSTRALIA
BY CAPRICORN LINK (AUSTRALIA) PTY. LTD.
P.O. BOX 704, WINDSOR, NSW 2756, AUSTRALIA

ISBN-13: 978-1-4027-3526-4

ISBN-10: 1-4027-3526-X

PRINTED AND BOUND IN THE U.S.A. BY MAPLE-VAIL

FOR INFORMATION ABOUT CUSTOM EDITIONS, SPECIAL SALES,
PREMIUM AND CORPORATE PURCHASES, PLEASE CONTACT
STERLING SPECIAL SALES DEPARTMENT AT 800-805-5489 OR
SPECIALSALES@STERLINGPUB.COM.

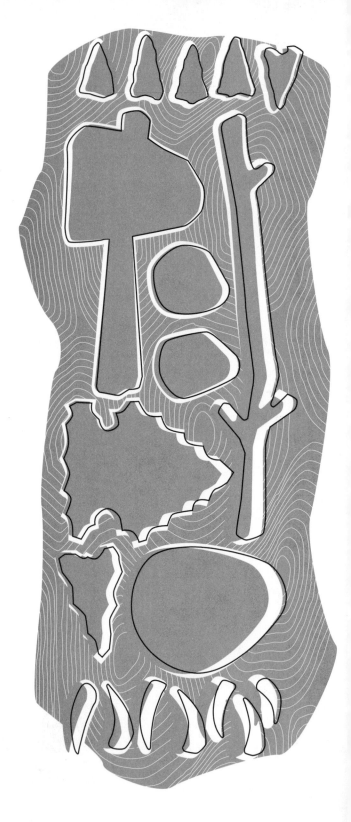

CONTENTS

CHAPTER 4

**DR. STRANGEGLOVE &
THE MEDICAL MYSTERY TOUR**   59

*You're not a doctor, you just play one
in this chapter. Here's the short course
on medical and health issues that arise
during pregnancy.*

CHAPTER 5

JUST THE TWO OF US   89

*You can still have a life during
pregnancy—even a sex life. This chapter
includes suggestions for strengthening
your relationship, from a workout for
two to sexual positions for the expectant
couple.*

CHAPTER 6

CAVEMAN COOKS FOR THREE (OR MORE)   113

*Learn kitchen basics and add the recipes
in this chapter to your repertoire.
Includes essential dietary and
nutritional information for mom-to-be
and baby.*

CHAPTER 7

THE NEONATAL NEANDERTHAL   171

*Here's how the whole birth thing might
unfold, from the first signs of labor to the
earth-shattering moment you first bring
Baby Unibrow home to the cave.*

Resources   209

Glossary   211

Index   221

Acknowledgments   234

CHAPTER 1

**CONGRATULATIONS!
NOW KISS THE STONE AGE GOODBYE**   1

*Here's the skinny on how this book
is going to save your Cro-Magnon
keister now that you're suddenly being
forced to evolve. Meet Gronk, your
tour guide, and get ready to assume a
more upright posture.*

CHAPTER 2

THE TIMES THEY ARE A-CHANGIN'   11

*What to expect when you're expecting is
change, and lots of it—this chapter will
help you deal with the transformations to
come. Includes a timeline of key moments
and milestones.*

CHAPTER 3

CAN-DO CAVEMAN   35

*Become a responsible, well prepared
parent-to-be in this chapter. Explore
ways to better yourself, identify habits
to drop and adopt, and fail-safe massage
techniques to use on your mate.*

CHAPTER 1

CONGRATULATIONS! NOW KISS THE STONE AGE GOODBYE

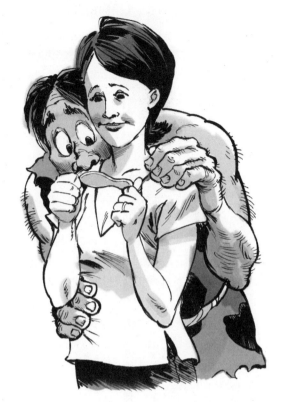

THE DOCTOR JUST made it official: you and your partner have a baby on the way. As a guy who hasn't been down this road before, you're probably a little slow to grasp exactly what it means to be "expectant." What it means, caveman, is that the mom-to-be will be expecting much more of you.

For the expectant mom, pregnancy can be a mental and physical roller coaster ride. With the joy, elation, and anticipation of pending parenthood, she must also contend with changing bodily proportions, a queasy stomach, and an ever-present urge to get horizontal—though not necessarily with you. Being pregnant in many cases means a vastly diminished ability to function full time at a reasonable capacity. Pregnant women need support so they can focus on the primary tasks at hand: nurturing a healthy baby through to term and delivering a healthy bundle of joy as quickly and painlessly as possible. The last thing they want or deserve is a knuckledragger who can't cope with the new demands of pregnancy and fatherhood. What they need is someone who's willing and able to evolve into a well prepared, secure partner, someone who's ready to stand upright and embrace all the new responsibilities of expectant fatherhood.

Well, Mr. Unibrow, that someone is you, the expectant father, the impregnator, the prehistoric procreator whose duties for the next nine months—and beyond—now include catering to your woman's needs and wants. Whether it's preparing and serving a nutritious, tasty meal when she's too tired to cook, delivering a timely massage when she's sore, uncomfortable, or tense, or engaging in a snuggle session when she needs some cuddling with her caveman, your time has come.

Besides attending to your pregnant woman in her time of need, you will be expected to take care of other baby-business, like getting your home ready, buying the right equipment, participating in pregnancy- and baby-related discussions and decisions with the mom-to-be, and being on call for what will seem like an endless procession of doctor visits.

That's right, men: when there's a bun in the oven, it's time to get your butt in gear.

Then there's the task of preparing yourself mentally (and physically) for the life-altering events that lie ahead. How will you reconcile your prehistoric proclivities with the realities of pregnancy? Can your psyche deal with your woman's changing physical dimensions and hormonally driven mood swings? Are you prepared to become her caterer, capable of churning out full meals at a moment's notice? Will you have the fortitude to witness—and actively participate in—the wonder of childbirth without smelling salts or prescription sedatives? Will you know a lullaby or two to sing to the newborn in your best caveman croon?

If these questions overwhelm your primitive sensibilities, you're not alone. When it comes to prenatal preparedness, especially among first-timers, much of the male species falls short. Thankfully, men are generally an adaptable bunch. When the situation—and our woman—demands it, we *can* evolve. And with the help of this book, you shall.

The pages that follow will coax the expectant father out of his cave and help him embrace the opportunity to develop into a full-fledged partner in pregnancy and a can-do Cro-Magnon caregiver. The goal is simple: to rid the father-to-be of that boar-in-the-headlights feeling by imparting him with the essentials to navigate this unfamiliar and potentially overwhelming environment.

Think you're not cut out to be a dad? All you need are a few primitive essentials to embark on the right course:

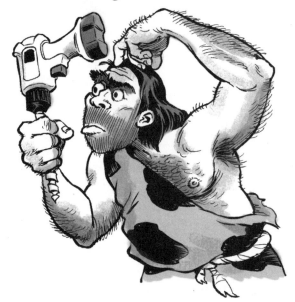

▶ Opposable thumbs and digits that move independently of one another

▶ Familiarity with a few rudimentary household tools and implements and the dexterity to handle them (clubs and other forms of cudgel excluded)

- The agility to hunt and gather household necessities, the means to transport them back to the cave, and the skill to assemble them if necessary

- The mental acuity to distinguish between a rattle and a rubber duck, a doctor and a doula

- Access to power sources—fire, electricity, and the like—and the sophistication to harness them safely

- A *tabula rasa* mindset in which you're open to learning new things and unlearning bad habits

- The curiosity to find out how other modern male *Homo sapiens* go about this fatherhood thing

- And most importantly, a desire to help the woman in your life when she needs it most

For expectant moms, this book is a ticket to freedom and goodwill during pregnancy. With a prehistoric partner who's helpful, handy, and proactive, she'll have more time for activities, exercise, and relaxation, three crucial ingredients for a healthy, less stressful pregnancy. It's tough enough to carry a growing baby for nine months. Expectant mothers would much rather be reading a book, taking a yoga class, or picking out the right shade of paint for the baby's nursery than laboring throughout pregnancy because the guy in her life is a Stone Age throwback, paralyzed by the thought of fatherhood.

Pregnancy means major life changes, but it needn't turn you into an indentured servant for the expectant mom. You still need to heed the call of your inner caveman by pursuing the Paleolithic pastimes you've always enjoyed. Your willingness to become a quality parent-in-waiting earns you that right.

It doesn't, however, give you the right to take leave of reality. So instead of curling up into the fetal position like your unborn child, why not rise to the challenge? You have much to gain and little to lose. Let your lady take a well-deserved seat on the couch, kick off her shoes, and watch as you evolve during the next three trimesters into a baby-ready cavedad-to-be. There will be plenty of time later to address your posture issues, personal grooming habits, and other Cro-Magnon tendencies. Now it's time to get down to some serious paternal and parental preparation.

WHY READ THIS BOOK?

There's a reason this book landed in your hands: because you or someone you know thought it would be a good idea for you to read it. Maybe you purchased it yourself, had it given to you as a gift, or had it slipped to you anonymously by your wife, your mother-in-law, another member of your clan, a neighbor, your family doctor, a golf buddy, a work colleague, or even the postal delivery person.

Think you're not the kind of guy who can benefit from reading a pregnancy and childbirth guide? Think again. Nine months is a long time, and you're going to need help along the way. Finally there's a pregnancy guidebook written by cavemen specifically for cavemen—guys with throwback tendencies who happen to have a child on the way. As a group, these cavedads-to-be represent no small segment of the male population. All the information and insights included in these pages are specially tuned to communicate with them on their unique wavelength. Because when it comes to communication skills, cavemen can have a pretty limited bandwidth.

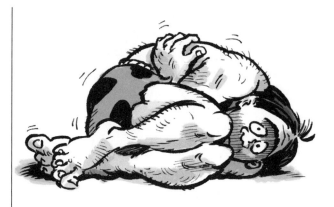

Not to worry. This is not a textbook that tests your attention span, nor is it an exhaustive, authoritative reference book that delves into and dwells on the minutiae of pregnancy and childbirth. Leave those tomes to the ladies. Here's a volume full of timely, practical, and accurate information and advice, written especially for the simpler segment of the human species. This book has illustrations, monosyllabic words, and bite-size pieces of information (plus a glossary at the end) to maximize the caveman's enjoyment and minimize the instances in which he stops, scratches his head, and mutters to his woman, "I don't get it."

To keep the expectant father's head from exploding, the material in this book addresses only pregnancy and childbirth. We know the caveman's capacity for processing new information is limited, especially on subjects of the magnitude discussed here, so the fatherhood stuff we'll save for another book. Not only have we filled the *Caveman's Pregnancy Companion* with the most up-to-date information and sage advice for the

period from conception to the day you bring cavebaby home, we've also laced it with a joke or two, because without the ability to laugh in the face of adversity and smile when you're stressed out, pregnancy and childbirth can become pretty overwhelming.

Even with your sense of humor intact, preparing for the arrival of a child is a mighty undertaking. But you're not in this by yourself. For support, you can rely on your pregnant partner, your parents, friends who have been down the pregnancy path before and lived to tell the tale, even professional counselors, whose advice often comes at an exorbitant hourly rate. These are the types of people who can talk you down off the proverbial pregnancy ledge and help you maintain perspective when things get particularly stressful or befuddling.

Fortunately, much of the pregnancy and childbirth advice and information you seek is contained right here in these pages, so you won't have to pay a bloated fee to obtain it. The fact is, much of what you read in this book is current, accurate information provided directly by doctors, nutritionists, massage therapists, educators, and other professionals specializing in prenatal and neonatal issues. From an expectant caveman's perspective, this is legitimately useful stuff.

Given the import medical and health issues carry throughout a woman's pregnancy, you will also hear a lot from our resident medical expert, **Dr. Brian**. A caveman and a family doctor in real life (apparently the two are not mutually exclusive), Dr. Brian weighs in with a medical perspective on a variety of issues the expectant couple likely will face as their pregnancy progresses. He touches on such topics as the mysterious couvade condition that seizes some men during pregnancy, the surprising benefits that Kegel exercises can offer both men and women, and the APGAR test that your child will take just moments after birth.

Also weighing in at various points of the book are two of our other resident experts and members of the Expectant Caveman's Ad Hoc Female Advisory Council: **Kelli**, a registered dietician and prenatal nutrition and dietary expert, and **Desirae**, a doula and prenatal massage therapist. These are women who know their stuff, so listen closely when they have a point to make.

Ponder This items also pop up throughout the book, helping fill in some of the gaping holes in the caveman's knowledge of the world of expectant parenthood by addressing a range of disparate topics, from an explanation of the strange pregnancy-related phenomenon known as the nesting instinct to an up-close-and-personal look at labor-and-delivery nurses.

CULTIVATING THE CAVEMAN

If their loping gait, furred digits, and oversize brows don't give them away, their approach to life certainly will. They are twenty-first-century Cro-Magnons, and even today millions of them walk among us, hoping to blend in with their natty attire, their high-tech communications devices, and their modern speech patterns.

Hidden behind that contemporary visage is a caveman crying out for help polishing his rough edges, a guy in desperate need of cultivation. He appears to move effortlessly in a world of golf foursomes, backyard barbecues, and shiny SUVs. But ultimately those modern accoutrements cannot hide the rustic habits and rudimentary social skills that make him immediately recognizable as a true caveman.

Does hearing this description cause the hair on your neck to stand on end? That's probably because it cuts a little too close to the bone. The truth is, you could very well be one of these neo-cavemen yourself. (The mere fact you have hair on your neck is a pretty strong indication that's the case.) But don't be ashamed of who you are. So what if your tastes, pursuits, and habits tend toward the unsophisticated? You are a man—albeit one to whom the theory of evolution does not necessarily apply.

As it turns out, many of the throwback qualities that make you a modern caveman may be what attracted your partner to you in the first place. And now the two of you are expecting a child. What happens when a Neanderthal like you is confronted with the reality of impending fatherhood? Really there are only two choices: you can bury your head in the sand and stubbornly cling to your Cro-Magnon ways; or you can embrace the life changes that lie ahead by changing your ways and shaping yourself into a father-to-be your partner will be proud of, thankful for, and reliant upon. This book is for the brave, responsible men who choose the latter route.

As a caveman living in the fast-paced twenty-first century, you may be driven by a peculiar urge to walk in the shoes of the more polished members of the male species. Maybe you are someone who is motivated to seek personal enrichment. Perhaps it's not your own internal curiosity or burning desire for self-improvement so much as external forces (read: the demands of your woman) that point you in new directions. Whatever the case, the bottom line is the same: you must evolve.

This book is written especially for the caveman who wants or needs cultivation— the guy who's ultimately destined to return to his cave, but not before becoming a better-equipped and motivated expectant father. It's for that huge contingent of the male populace who believe:

- The term "hairdo" applies to the entire body

- The idea of stovetop cooking is warming his hands over the burner

- The idea of a vegetarian meal is a lip full of chewing tobacco

- Yoga is either a creamy dairy product or a wizened Jedi master

When the situation calls for a caveman to adapt, either out of necessity or curiosity, this is a book you'll rely upon to make the process less painful, even rewarding, enlightening and—dare we say?—enjoyable.

SENSITIVE GUYS: YOUR ROLE MODELS

When it comes to pregnancy and the idea of impending fatherhood, the cavemen of today can be an impressionable, gullible lot, easily misled and misinformed by false wisdom passed down from one male generation to the next.

Maybe you've been led to believe that, like most males throughout the animal kingdom (and many of your *Homo sapiens* homeboys), your involvement in the child-rearing process ends at the moment of conception. But as a human being living here in the twenty-first century, you're not getting off the hook that easy. The fatherhood role you've seen reinforced in all those *Leave It to Beaver* reruns has changed. Ward Cleaver is a dinosaur. Thus the expectant caveman needs to look elsewhere for his role models, and (speaking of beavers) the animal kingdom is a good place to start. Nature is full of examples of males seizing control of childbearing and child-rearing responsibilities. Did you know, for example, that males in 90 percent of bird species provide some form of parental care, while the males in some species of fish mind the nest and the eggs inside it? As an expectant father, these are the males you should emulate. Here are a few other examples of males going above and beyond the call of duty during and after pregnancy:

- **Male seahorses** embrace fatherhood. They carry the eggs and bear full child-rearing responsibilities once the eggs hatch.

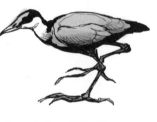

- The **male jacana bird** is a true stud. Not only does he bear responsibility for incubating eggs and raising the young, he's also forced to patient-

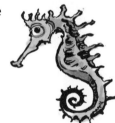

ly sit on the eggs and watch while the mother bird copulates with other males right under her mate's beak.

- The **giant water bug male** is no stranger to heavy parental burdens. His duties begin when a female attaches herself to him and cements as many as 150 eggs onto his back. The female departs promptly after unburdening herself, leaving the male to carry the load for the next month, during which time the eggs will triple in size.

- His name might not imply it, but the **male Panamanian poison-arrow frog** is one sensitive amphibian. He sits on the eggs and keeps them hydrated with moisture from his skin. Once the tadpoles have hatched, he carries them on his back to water.

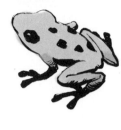

- Who wears the pants in the **emperor penguin**'s family? Tough to say. The male is responsible for incubating his mate's egg. While he's doing this inland, his mate returns to the sea to feed. When the egg hatches, he produces a type of regurgitated food called "penguin milk" for the new chick.

- The **male red fox** is the consummate gentleman when it comes to treating his vixen right. He supplies her with fresh food several times a day while she nurses the young ones.

These are the organisms with which you will soon become kindred spirits, your role models in the months ahead as you embark on your prenatal journey.

THE FRUITS OF YOUR LABOR

Well, Rick is the kind of man that...Well, if I were a woman...I should be in love with Rick. But what a fool I am talking to a beautiful woman about another man.

—CAPTAIN RENAULT, CASABLANCA

You're scratching your beguiled head, wondering, "What's in this for me?" After all, we are creatures driven by self-interest. Why should you invest the time and energy to become a full partner during pregnancy? Your caveman ways have served you well to this point, so why change now?

As any caveman who's been through the rigors of pregnancy and childbirth can attest, making the effort to be a well prepared, eminently competent father-to-be comes with many fringe benefits. Most importantly, by turning yourself into a more responsible and responsive member of the household and your woman's pregnancy partner, you'll be much better equipped for the lifelong parenting journey that lies ahead, with skills, habits, and qualities you can adapt and apply to all facets of your life. Like Humphrey Bogart's character Rick in *Casablanca*, you'll become the kind of guy men want to be and women want to be with—not that the thought of being with another woman ever crosses your mind before, during, or after pregnancy.

Here are a few of the other perks you're destined to enjoy when you join the exclusive company of highly evolved cave-dads-to-be:

PERK 1: The goodwill you show toward your woman during pregnancy should make her more open to your requests, more willing to fulfill your needs, and generally more pliable. Women have long memories. Your learning new skills should translate into many long-term benefits.

PERK 2: You'll exude an unspoken but clear sense of confidence that comes from the knowledge of the finer points of being a responsible and proactive expectant parent. Your skills as a highly competent parent-to-be will be a source of personal pride, a true accomplishment, and a demonstration of your mental aptitude, perseverance, and ability to perform under pressure. You are a can-do caveman.

PERK 3: Your status as an expectant father brings you good karma. A lucrative bonus may unexpectedly come your way at work. Your golf handicap may drop. The bald spot on the top of your head may begin to grow hair again. You could develop an uncanny ability to locate empty parking spaces quickly. You may even surprise your mate and yourself with newfound prowess as a lover.

PERK 4: You'll discover that an improved diet, more exercise, and a purging of bad habits translate into a clearer complexion, sounder sleep patterns, a fitter figure, and (you hope) a more upright posture.

PERK 5: Some perks you may not necessarily clamor for, but doing what it takes to be a responsible cavedad-to-be is apt to get you noticed. Even your in-laws will view you as a superstar. Always wanted to be the apple of your mother-in-law's eye or hear your father-in-law use the phrase "Why can't you be more like [insert your name here]?" Here's your chance to shine.

PERK 6: An absentee dad-to-be you are not. You're a full partner in the Babymaking Inc. joint venture you and your woman formed together, not just the inseminator and the hunter-gatherer. Sure, you'll share in some of the extra work and angst associated with pregnancy. But you'll also share more in the rewards, gaining an emotional stake in the health of your baby and family, plus more intimacy with your partner.

PERK 7: You and your woman will find new common ground, working out side by side on the elliptical machine, debating the relative merits of various parenting strategies, watching food shows on TV, discussing potential interior decorating approaches for the nursery, maybe even going to the spa together for a waxing (go early, it takes a long time for the full-body treatment).

MEET GRONK

The need inside you, I see it showin'
Whoa, the seed inside ya, baby, do you feel
*   it growin'?*
Are you happy you know it? That you're...
Havin' my baby
— PAUL ANKA, "(YOU'RE) HAVING MY BABY"

Even the most resourceful cavemen cannot survive in unfamiliar, sometimes hostile territory on instincts alone. That's why automobiles now come equipped with GPS systems.

Unfortunately, a GPS system is of no help to expectant fathers when it comes to finding one's way in the prenatal wilderness. What the cavedad-to-be needs is a mentor, a throwback like him who bravely and successfully navigated the pregnancy path and who emerged on the other side a changed man after the birth of his child.

Enter **Gronk**, a caveman like you and the guy who will serve as your personal guide for the next forty weeks (which, incidentally, is the typical gestation period for a fetus inside the womb). If you are anything like Gronk, you want to believe you are self-sufficient enough not to need handholding to cope with and embrace the demands, expectations, responsibilities, milestones, and amazing moments that come during pregnancy and childbirth. Don't be deceived. The environment you are entering can be unforgiving to the uninitiated or unprepared—especially so for caveman types who have trouble wrapping their minds around such things as

GRONK: UP CLOSE AND PERSONAL

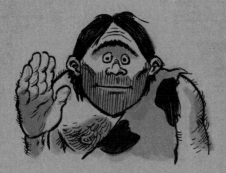

BORN: Sometime in the 1970s, in a meadow by a stream

BACKGROUND: Father, Grulk, is a mason; mother, Lucy, is an anthropologist; oldest of three children; sister Fern, brother Durk; college graduate (alma mater undisclosed)

PROFESSION: Sales (construction materials)

HOBBIES: Playing drums; hunting; taxidermy; softball; reading the Sunday comics

TURN-ONS: Macrobrew (preferably in the can) and women who drink it; weather; blackjack; classic rock and hip-hop played loud; going barefoot; the sound of wind rustling the trees

TURN-OFFS: Duplicitous people; wearing ties; high-pitched sounds; books without pictures

FAVORITE SONGS: "Ballad of the Caveman" by Oingo Boingo; anything by Queens of the Stone Age

FAVORITE TV SHOWS: *The Flintstones*; *Land of the Lost*; any show featuring Claymation characters

ROLE MODELS: John Belushi; John "Bonzo" Bonham; *Homo habilis;* Oetzi the Neolithic Iceman

GOALS: To be a good partner during pregnancy and a good father to his children; to learn a second language (and get better at the first); to shave less; to finally finish building that beer-can pyramid after eight long years

complex emotions, new responsibilities, and the cryptic assembly instructions accompanying baby-related equipment.

Gronk will serve as your mentor, walking beside you on the sometimes tortuous pregnancy path detailed in the pages that follow. Think of him as the GPS you can turn to for direction during your woman's pregnancy, the one who will take your hairy palm in his to guide you on this journey as you evolve from a potential pregnancy train wreck into a competent, confident, and compliant cavedad-to-be.

As you'll learn from your own experiences and by following Gronk through the pages of this book, the evolutionary process is not always going to be easy. In fact, it might get downright painful at times as you shed old habits in favor of new ones, take on new responsibilities, develop new skills, and tap into emotions both masculine and feminine you never knew existed.

You may waver in your belief that you can live up to the expectations facing a father-to-be. But remember, cavemen like us have been doing the pregnancy and childbirth thing for thousands of years, often in a highly capable manner. Somehow, the human race has managed to persevere and multiply. But as a caveman whose shortcomings are well documented, you'll need Gronk's help to become fit to survive—and thrive—during and after your woman's pregnancy.

So don't be stubborn or bashful. Slip your hand into Gronk's and let's get this journey of prenatal discovery and personal enrichment underway.

CHAPTER 2

THE TIMES THEY ARE A-CHANGIN'

*Her point was that there was too much
love and beauty for just the two of us....
And every day we kept a child out of the
world was a day he might later regret
having missed.*

—H.I. McDUNNOUGH, *RAISING ARIZONA*

N A WINDSWEPT PLAIN somewhere in the countryside of what is now the city of Heidelberg in southwest Germany, a faint light flickers in a deep rock recess partially hidden by a thicket of overgrown vines and bushes.

A faint light also flickers in the mind of a Cro-Magnon male who, along with the rest of his clan, dwells in the space beyond this narrow mouth in the rock. This is the place he, his woman, and a multigenerational tribe of their relatives call home. And by the prevailing standards of some 20,000 years

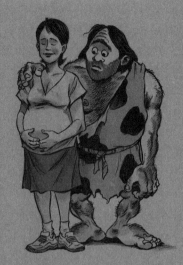

GROW WITH GRONK

What the caveman stands to gain
from reading Chapter 2:

▶ **AN UNDERSTANDING** of the emotional swings and feelings of ambivalence that may affect both expectant parents

▶ **AN IDEA** of how the nine months of pregnancy might unfold, from key milestones to major developmental moments inside the womb

▶ **A GRASP** of the physical and mental demands of expectant parenthood

▶ **A KNOWLEDGE** of how hormones may affect a woman during pregnancy

▶ **STRATEGIES** for relieving stress, releasing tension, and savoring time together and independent of your mate

▶ **STRATEGIES** for lessening the baby-related financial burden

▶ **INSIGHTS** on ways an expectant father can stay true to his caveman self

ago, it isn't a bad place; plenty of reindeer skins and small game pelts to keep things cozy, several goats meandering about, a huge array of stone tools, an impressive arsenal of spears and clubs, a colorful collection of cave paintings on the walls, plus a fire to provide light and warmth to the dank space.

On this day the middle-aged Cro-Magnon male, all seventeen years of him, sits close beside his fourteen-year-old mate, appearing dazed, a little perturbed, but mostly confused. Through a series of rudimentary syllables, facial expressions, and emphatic gestures, he has just learned from his woman that she expects her womb to bear fruit in some moons' time.

His prominent jaw has gone slack and his high forehead is furrowed with wrinkles. The Cro-Magnon shifts his thousand-mile stare to the paintings on the walls surrounding him. He sees scenes depicting men hurling spears, felling and skinning large mammals, copulating with multiple partners, climbing trees, scaling cliffs, dancing around bonfires, and playing crude instruments. He wonders if siring an offspring will put an end to the activities he enjoys so much. His imagination swims with possibilities, some tantalizing, some petrifying. Will his woman and child survive the rigors of childbirth? Will he? Will he be able to provide for the needs of a child—food, shelter, a warm and safe place to sleep? Will the baby be a male or female? Will it resemble him or perhaps look like one of the gods he worships, with the head of a horse, the horns of a ram, or the tail of a giant cat? What will they call the newborn? And when will the child be able to join him for the hunt?

For this man of the Pleistocene epoch and for scores of cavemen who walk among us today, the ambivalence of pending parenthood is a difficult emotion to process. His facial expressions alternate between a smile and a grimace. In need of some crisp Pleistocene air to collect his thoughts, the Cro-Magnon nods to his woman, grabs his fur cloak and spear, then exits the cave, resolved to climb his "thinking tree" for some alone time.

Strikingly similar domestic scenes have played out in hominid and *Homo sapiens* households for hundreds of centuries. And they continue to play out today as moms- and dads-to-be wrestle with the ambivalent feelings of pending parenthood. It's natural for expectant parents to experience conflicting emotions as the birth of a child approaches, even if it took them awhile to get pregnant in the first place. If you and your woman are like most parents-to-be, there will come a moment during the pregnancy when the two of you ask yourselves the question expectant parents have been scratching their heads about virtually since the last Ice Age: "Are we doing the right thing having a baby?" That question inevitably leads to another: "Do I—and do we—have what it takes to be good parents?"

Rest assured those two questions will resurface numerous times, not only during pregnancy but throughout your life as a parent as well. Ambivalence, apprehension, and insecurity are common emotions for adults during the long and winding road of the childbearing and childrearing years. But ask most parents and they'll tell you the high points of pregnancy and parenting easily overshadow any misgivings or doubts that surface at particularly stressful moments. They'll also tell you that by trusting and acting upon your instincts, seeking advice from people you trust—friends, family, and pros who should know, such as doctors, nurses, and doulas—and reading books such as this, you can confidently answer those two time-worn questions in the affirmative.

Now is not the time to dwell too much on what might lie ahead for the two of you as parents. Sure, you will spend many idle moments in the months to come daydreaming about how life might unfold for the three of you. But there will be plenty of time later to ride the parental roller coaster. For roughly the next forty weeks, you will be strapped into a different thrill ride known as pregnancy. Making it through that ride with your wits and your relationship intact should be your primary focus. How you fare during those nine months will go a long way toward determining whether you and your woman ultimately opt to buy a ticket for another spin on the baby tilt-a-whirl. But let's not get ahead of ourselves.

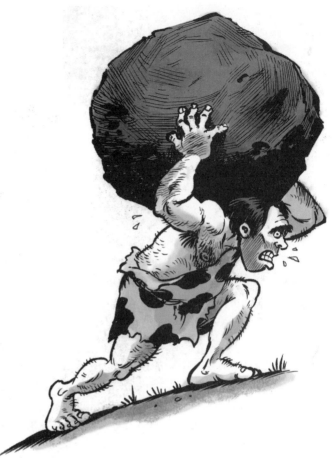

Someday, when you and your woman are considering whether to have another child, the two of you will look back on this pregnancy and wonder, "How exactly did we spend those nine months?" You were busy enough before a baby entered the picture. Now, besides holding down your jobs and attending to your normal day-to-day responsibilities, the two of you have a pregnancy, a gestating fetus, and pending parenthood to think about.

The time leading up to the birth of your first child can become a blur if you don't make a point of slowing down to savor what will be the last months, weeks, and days you experience as a childless person (if this is your first child). Here's where a caveman's extra-keen olfactory sense comes in handy, for you will need it to stop and smell the roses during pregnancy, savoring the high points and helping one another through the low ones.

A woman who is pregnant for the first time is known as a "primigravida." As her male counterpart, you are simply called "primitive," "primordial," or "primeval." For a couple of "primis" like the two of you, it would be nice to know exactly when the high and low points of pregnancy might occur so you can prepare for them ahead of time.

However, that's not usually possible. The nine months of pregnancy unfold differently for every couple. Some partners sail through gestation with nary a complication, effortlessly passing those forty weeks as if it were their ninth child, not their first. Other couples encounter difficulties virtually from Day One, be it health issues, emotional obstacles, or a combination of the two. For some, time seems to accelerate during the prenatal period. For others, it seems to stand still.

For the two of you, chances are the prenatal experience will fall somewhere between those extremes. One day you may feel fully prepared to tackle the duties of expectant fatherhood and the next you may feel utterly overwhelmed by those responsibilities. One moment your woman may brighten a room with her pregnant-woman glow and the next

she may turn the same room green with the intensity of her nausea.

Such is life on the stomach-churning, mind-scrambling prenatal roller coaster. Indeed, pregnancy is largely about dealing with the unexpected. But while there's no predicting just what will transpire in the months leading up to the birth of a child, there are certain things you and your woman can expect to happen, a long procession of milestones to savor, obstacles to overcome, deadlines to meet, dates to anticipate and dread, and achievements to reflect upon.

With a baby on the way, an expectant couple's mindset and priorities begin to change rapidly. If this breakneck evolutionary pace is enough to at times overwhelm the typically composed, prepared female half of the partnership, imagine what it might do to an uninitiated and unprepared caveman. It's enough to make a grown man crawl back to his bed of leaves and twigs and bury his head.

Here's a chapter designed to help expectant fathers avoid those breakdowns by shedding light on some of the major developments that lie ahead for both of you—the physical, mental, and emotional markers that are sure to make the months to come some of the most interesting and challenging you are ever likely to experience. All sorts of surprises are crouching along the pregnancy path, waiting to ambush the two of you as you pass. If you're clued in to those surprises beforehand, you stand a much better chance of reaching the end of the path relatively unscathed.

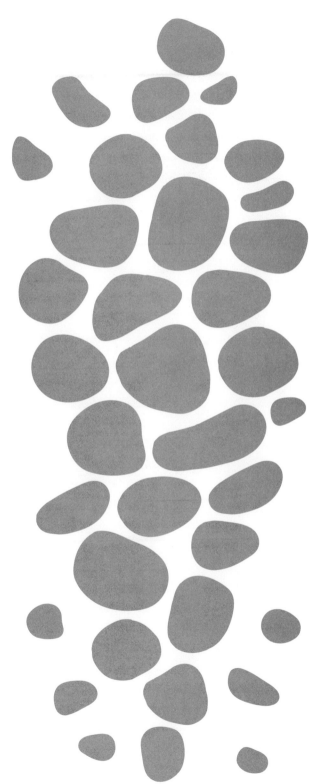

STRANGER IN A
STRANGE LAND

*Never in my sweet, short life
Have I felt like this before*

—THE ROLLING STONES, "NO EXPECTATIONS"

As a creature for whom abstract thought is elusive, as one who finds comfort in the familiar, the modern caveman's first instinct in attempting to grasp the proportions of the situation in which he is about to be plunged is to scour his memory in search of something in his past that might compare with expectant fatherhood. His search comes up empty.

He does recall, however, that the last time he felt so powerless was as an 18-year-old college fraternity pledge. But if Mr. Alpha Knucka Dragga thought being a pledge was challenging, wait until he gets a dose of pregnancy and childbirth. In some respects, as shown in the "Fraternal and Paternal Rites of Passage" grid on the following page, being a father-in-waiting is like being a fraternity brother-in-waiting, minus the close encounters with sheep. The bottom line, however, is that attaining fatherhood is serious stuff; attaining brotherhood was merely some weird male bonding dance.

FRATERNAL AND PATERNAL RITES OF PASSAGE

	THE PLEDGE	THE "PRIMI" MALE
NEW NAME	Monkeyboy	Honey-do
WORKING TO EARN PASSAGE TO	Brotherhood	Fatherhood
TO WHOM HE MUST ANSWER	Fifty frat boys	One pregnant woman (and sometimes her mother)
PRIMARY RESPONSIBILITIES	Fetching drinks; absorbing useless fraternity facts; submitting to senseless acts for the entertainment of others; becoming a worthy brother	Procuring household supplies; performing constructive baby-oriented tasks; accepting reality; subjugating one's needs to the greater good of the couple; becoming a worthy expectant father
REASON(S) FOR ALTERED SLEEP HABITS	Late-night drinking games; attempting to learn a semester's worth of material in one night of studying	Stress; attempting to complete a decade's worth of home tasks in nine months
MAIN SOURCE(S) OF STRESS	Approaching exam in class he has yet to attend	Approach of one of life's biggest tests: parenthood
MEANS OF STRESS RELIEF	Binge drinking	Binge eating
SACRIFICES HE WILL BE ASKED TO MAKE	Time with girlfriend; academics; healthy diet, liver	Unfettered access to guys-only recreational activities (golf, etc.); vices (smoking, gambling, etc.)
PAIN HE MUST ENDURE	Paddling, branding, dry-heaving	Physical and mental withdrawal from vices; saying yes when what he really means is no
LIFE LESSONS LEARNED ALONG THE WAY	That excessive alcohol consumption interferes with life goals; that any daughter of yours won't come within a hundred yards of a fraternity house	That an excessive focus on the self interferes with family goals; that life changes don't mean life as you know it has ended; that carrying and giving birth to a baby are truly heroic acts
REWARD(S) FOR COMPLETING JOURNEY	The bond of brotherhood, heavyweight drinking skills; ability to make a toga from a bedsheet with no safety pins	Life with a beautiful child and a wonderful family

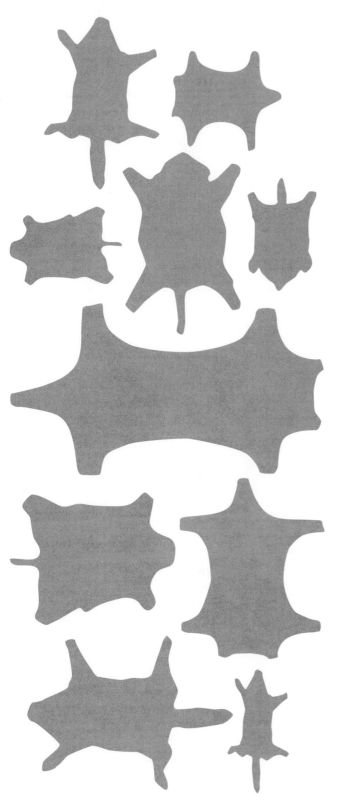

EMBRYONIC JOURNEY: MOMENTOUS GESTATIONAL MOMENTS, MONTH BY MONTH

You are in for an action-packed forty weeks. Besides the many mental and physical issues parents-to-be must confront, there are concerns associated with pregnancy, as well as considerations related to home, family, finances, even pets.

The following timelines chronicle some of the key milestones and moments you, expectant mom, and baby are likely to encounter in the months to come, broken down by trimester and by month. Each timeline encompasses a thirteen-week period, approximately the length of a trimester. Keep in mind, however, the pregnancy you share with your partner may unfold nothing like the chronologies in the pages that follow.

THE FIRST TRIMESTER

	FIRST MONTH	SECOND MONTH	THIRD MONTH
BABY	Embryo is implanted in the lining of uterus and nourished by mother Heart is beating and limb buds begin to grow	Embryo developing super rapidly: lungs, brain, stomach, and other organs are online and growing Head, eyes, hands, feet, and digits are recognizable	Baby looks "human" but with extra long arms and big head Genitals forming and recognizable
BABY SIZE	Ladybug (¼")	Grape (1⅛")	Golf-club head (2½–3", ½–1 oz)
HER	Joy, anxiety, worry Surging hormonal activity Breasts become tender	Nausea and fatigue Food cravings for protein Aversion to onions and other strong flavors and smells	Really pooped, spends more time in prone position Need to pee in the middle of the night: 2 times Breasts grow in size and stature
CAVEMAN	Quits tobacco habit cold turkey Considers "planning" an afternoon on the couch	Couvade symptoms start (see p. 24): nausea, breasts and waistline swell Feeling a little overwhelmed: let's try the fetal position	Cold showers part of daily routine Focus on actual planning, now
COUPLE	At-home pregnancy test taken (twice) and it's positive! "Omigod, are we ready?!" Make first of many lists of questions for doctor	Mood swings become an issue Sexual activity falls off What's the insurance situation?	Embark on joint exercise routine Tell the world about the baby
HOMEFRONT	Shock and awe	Nesting instinct kicks in	Planning those home projects
DOCTOR	Make OB-GYN appointment for next month (6 weeks from test)	Confirmation! Bun is definitely in oven Due date calculation Full lab work done Discuss miscarriage issues and information	First trimester screening offered CVS (see p. 72) may be recommended Ultrasound may be ordered if due date is uncertain

THE SECOND TRIMESTER

	FOURTH MONTH	FIFTH MONTH	SIXTH MONTH
BABY	Eyebrows, eyelashes, and other hair growth begins Begins to pee, sleep, and kick Largely reduced chance of miscarriage	Makes faces (grimaces, smiles), sucks thumb, and swallows Teeth forming beneath gums Body is covered in waxy protective coating (vernix caseosa)	Opens eyes for the first time Begins to "explore the space" by moving around much more Female babies develop ovaries
BABY SIZE	Softball (6½–7", 6–7 oz)	Coconut (8–10", 1 lb)	Trout (11–14", 13/4–2 lb)
HER	Feeling baby movements Indigestion and heartburn Gained about 5 lb (more or less) Kegels, Kegels, Kegels (see p. 112)	Maternity clothes now a must Feels more energetic Hormones regain some balance Breasts start producing colostrum	Aversion to red meat, "I want ice cream!" Need to pee in the middle of the night: 4 times Pregnancy "glow" in full effect
CAVEMAN	Signs of competency as a cook Protective instincts surging "She's actually horny all the time!!"	Consults Cava Sutra for creative sexual input (see p. 96) First mental breakdown	Cooking tasty meals for mate with regularity Exercise regimen shows solid results; drops an inch from his waist size
COUPLE	Sexual relations improve Start prenatal massage routine	Enroll in parenting/birthing class Yoga together is actually fun	Too pooped for sex most of the time Tour the birthing facility
HOMEFRONT	Money worries and credit card balance may start to swell	Baby shower windfall	Vehicle prep, time for a better/bigger car?
DOCTOR	Should be able to hear fetal heart Ultrasound appointment, may be able to see sex of baby	Second trimester screening offered Amniocentesis (see p. 72) may be recommended Ultrasound may be ordered to assess fetal anatomy	Check blood pressure and weight Routine testing of urine

THE THIRD TRIMESTER

	SEVENTH MONTH	**EIGHTH MONTH**	**NINTH MONTH**
BABY	Fingernails and toenails growing May react to light and sounds from outside the womb Looks like a skinny little newborn—starting to fatten up for the big day	Gaining weight quickly Shifting and turning head more down toward the exit (cervix) Cries, hiccups	Lungs are mature and baby is fattening up ½ lb a week Things are getting cramped in there, baby is more curled up in "fetal position" Bones are hardening but skull is flexible in order to make it through the birth canal
BABY SIZE	Pot roast (14–16", 2½–3 ½ lb)	Football (16½–18", 4–6 lb)	Baby (19–20", 7–7 ½ lb)
HER	"Nothing fits me!" Blood pressure up slightly Constipation	Now must rely on sense of touch to tie shoes Takes to frequent snacking—no room for full meals Need to pee in the middle of the night: 5 times	Braxton Hicks contractions more frequent Walking getting a little tougher Feet swell Hard to get comfortable
CAVEMAN	Takes last "man" trip for foreseeable future Takes a practice run with the baby jogger Periodically ousted to sleep on couch or guest room	Planning route to hospital Practicing bedside manner	"Jumpstart labor sex" is a good thing (see p. 98) Calm and supportive
COUPLE	Infant CPR course Make postpartum childcare plans	Spend last long weekend away together Graduate from birthing/parenting class	Get serious about baby names Prepare birth announcements Pack that bag for the hospital
HOMEFRONT	Nursery work nearly complete	Dog and cat off to the vet for a check-up	Freezer full of caveman-prepared meals Mother-in-law moving in
DOCTOR	Have the circumcision discussion Glucose challenge test for gestational diabetes	Begin bi-weekly visits to OB-GYN Choose a pediatrician Preregister at the hospital Discuss preterm labor	Culture for GBS (see p. 81) Regular visits Call when your water breaks

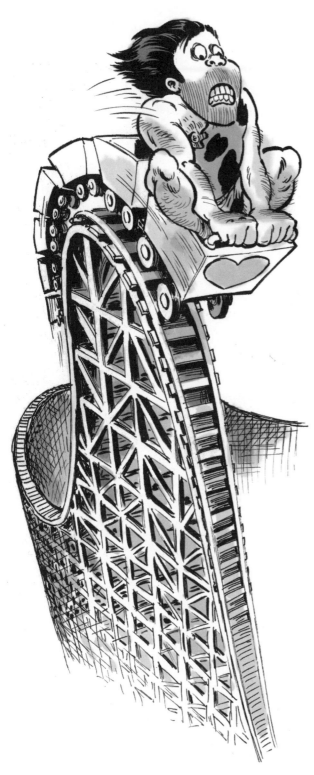

LOVE ROLLER COASTER

It's a mistake for which women have been chastising and punishing men for millennia: discounting or dismissing the genuineness of a woman's emotions and attributing her authentic feelings to inexplicable forces dwelling within. During pregnancy, or even more commonly during a woman's menstrual cycle, the Neolithic ninny may attempt to explain his partner's emotional behavior away the same way his caveman father did, and exactly as his caveman ancestors had done for eons before that. "It's just her time of the month," he says.

Few phrases a guy can utter evoke such a fast, furious response from a woman and get a guy into the doghouse quicker—not just because he has emotionally disenfranchised her (and made an oaf of himself) with one sentence, but because he is downright mistaken. Once punished for uttering those words, men who have the acuity to learn from their mistakes will never again use the phrase, even if it is exactly what they are thinking. Among the more thick-skulled members of the male species, however, it takes a few stays in the doghouse before he learns to bite his tongue. Some stone-headed Neanderthals never learn, though, and thus the misconception is perpetuated from one generation of cavemen to the next.

It is virtually impossible to definitively pin a pregnant person's behavior on hormones alone. While hormones may indeed be a major contributor to her emotional upheaval, that doesn't make what she's feeling and expressing any less genuine. This is how her true self is feeling and acting at the moment, so accept it or risk feeling her wrath. Cavemen prefer their explanations of things to be like jerky: cut and dried. But not all human behaviors and emotions, nor all pregnancy-related behavioral and emotional phenomena, are simple or easy to explain.

As you will soon discover if you haven't already, that holds true for both men and women. In the woman's case, it's neat and tidy for the caveman to attribute her mood swings during pregnancy solely to the hormonal upheaval her body is hosting. His first instinct is to oversimplify matters with a blanket statement.

The well-informed father-to-be knows better than to fall prey to such a trap. As we will discuss in a moment, it is true that changes in levels of such hormones as estrogen and progesterone when she's with child can indeed contribute to mood changes. But other issues not directly related to hormones are as important a factor in causing an expectant mother's emotional tides to behave unpredictably. Pregnancy-related physical symptoms like back pain, nausea, and swelling, as well as interrupted sleep, fatigue, body image issues, and general stress or tension, can have behavioral manifestations.

No matter how hard you want to find a straightforward explanation, it ultimately is impossible to separate the factors that contribute to mood changes. In fact, expectant fathers may be as prone to riding the emotional roller coaster as expectant mothers. With a child on the way, men, like women, may experience elevated stress, disrupted sleep patterns, fatigue, even the physical ailments associated with the mysterious condition known as couvade (see Dr. Brian, p. 24) that strikes some dads-to-be. Thus, guys, too, are prone to unpredictable moods when their woman is with child.

We commonly label these as "swings," but that may be a misnomer. Unlike with the swing of a pendulum, there is no predictable arc to an expectant parent's emotional path. Gut-wrenching plunges from high points to low, plus unexpected and sometimes drastic twists and turns, make the experience much more like riding a roller coaster blindfolded. In more isolated cases with pregnant women, the lows may lead to depression. In fact, recent medical research shows that depression with women may be more common during pregnancy (antepartum) than after delivery (postpartum).[1]

Here's where the caveman's powers of observation can be valuable. If you notice your woman's mood issues are especially pronounced—prolonged mood changes, sadness, frequent crying, sleep disturbance, expressing feelings of worthlessness—she may be suffering from clinical depression. Encourage her to (and if need be, gently insist that she) speak with her health care provider about

1. EVANS, J., JON HERON, AND HELEN FRANCOMB. Cohort study of depressed mood during pregnancy and after childbirth. http://bmj.bmjjournals.com/cgi/content/abstract/323/7307/257 (accessed 2001).

how she's feeling. It may be that the condition is treatable with counseling and/or medication that your woman's doctor deems safe for her to take during pregnancy.

THE HORMONAL HIGHWAY

We've established that one should never, ever be the first to blame a woman's mood changes on hormones. However, if she acknowledges to you that, yes, she's feeling crabby and it's probably due to hormones, only then can you also acknowledge the same connection, doing so without a hint of revelry or vindication in your voice.

The female body relies heavily on hormones to help regulate its functions during pregnancy (indeed, hormones are important messengers for male and female bodies, pregnant and otherwise). And while they aren't the sole contributor to mood swings, there is no denying their power to affect a pregnant woman's physical and emotional states, as well as fetal development. Hormones have been shown to contribute to headaches, backaches, fatigue, and other common conditions that periodically haunt some women during pregnancy.

A handful of hormones play particularly important roles in the expectant mom's body functions and the growth of the baby inside her. They include:

▶ **ESTROGEN.** Produced by the ovaries and later by the placenta, estrogen levels increase sharply when the woman's egg is fertilized. It's a powerful hormone that, like its counterpart testosterone, has gained renown for its role—real or imagined—in shaping relationships between the sexes through the ages. Estrogen has a definite role in pregnancy-related changes to a variety of interesting parts of the female anatomy, including the uterus, cervix, vagina, and breasts. After childbirth, a rapid change in estrogen levels is widely believed to be a cause for postpartum depression.

▶ **HUMAN CHORIONIC GONADOTROPIN,** HCG for short, is the hormone most early pregnancy tests seek to detect because it can be identified in urine. It comes from cells from the fertilized egg and prompts the ovaries to produce more estrogen and progesterone after conception.

▶ Like HCG, **HUMAN PLACENTAL LACTOGEN,** or HPL, is produced in the placenta. Its main job during pregnancy is to help the baby grow. It accomplishes that by sending messages that change the woman's metabolism and cause her body to divert crucial sugars and proteins to the baby. It also prepares her breasts for milk production.

▶ **OXYTOCIN.** Produced at low levels throughout pregnancy, oxytocin output increases during labor. A synthetic form of oxytocin known as Pitocin often may be administered in the hospital by members of the labor and delivery team to get the labor ball rolling.

DR. BRIAN

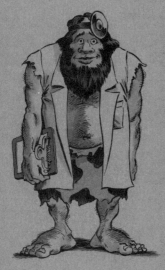

KING OF PAIN:
THE MYSTERY OF COUVADE

There's feeling her pain, then there's *living* her pain. Couvade—a term derived from the French word *couver*, which means "to hatch"—is a syndrome that takes male empathy with a woman's physical travails during pregnancy to the extreme. Expectant fathers afflicted with this mysterious phenomenon experience a "sympathetic pregnancy," exhibiting what are called "somatic" symptoms that cannot be explained physiologically but rather are physical manifestations of emotional issues. Symptoms of couvade (pronounced koo-vodd) may include indigestion, nausea and vomiting, weight gain, back pain, headaches, and more; they tend to take hold in the first trimester and worsen as pregnancy progresses. Then, just as inexplicably, they usually resolve when the child is born. All manner of psychological theories have been posited about the cause of couvade syndrome. One theory: it's the caveman's eccentric way of crying out for attention.

▶ **PROGESTERONE.** Here's another hormone produced by the ovaries and, further into pregnancy, by the placenta. Progesterone levels increase dramatically as the woman's body, realizing there is now a new baby on board, sends itself a signal to stop ovulating. From a medical perspective, a higher level of progesterone may cause fatigue and shortness of breath. Among its functions are keeping the uterus from contracting and promoting growth of uterine blood vessels that deliver nourishment to the baby. As with estrogen, its reduced presence after birth is linked to postpartum depression.

Armed with knowledge of how hormones fit into the broader behavioral picture during pregnancy, the caveman can better understand what's causing his woman to behave differently than what he's accustomed to. When she exhibits energetic bliss one hour and listless dejection the next, hormones may be one of several contributing factors. When she goes weeks spending long stretches of the day prone on the couch, then suddenly returns to her old, energetic self, he will know there are mysterious forces at work. He just won't know exactly which ones. And when he himself quickly goes from one moment feeling exhilarated and ready to accept the challenge of approaching fatherhood to the next feeling exhausted and overwhelmed by the thought of having a child, he will know he's riding the emotional mindscrambler.

STRESS RELIEF: DEFUSING THE TICKING TIME BOMB

It's been an especially harried week for the stressed-out couple. Both are facing high-pressure situations at work. While pursuing a painting project at home, the caveman discovers his basement is riddled with asbestos. To make matters worse, after yet another engine fire, the classic 1971 AMC Gremlin he's had since high school appears to be on its last legs. On top of that, his couvade-like back pains are really flaring up (see p. 24). Meanwhile, every item of clothing the expectant mom tries on no longer fits. Periodically she's too nauseous to eat when she knows she should be eating for two. Her parents have actually suggested moving into the basement apartment at least for a few months, and she seems open to the idea.

Tensions in the pregnant household are running high. Tempers and patience are short. Even the dog is avoiding you, sensing your foul mood. And there the two of you go again, asking yourselves that question: Are we doing the right thing, having a baby? The answer, of course, is moot; you're having a child in a matter of months, regardless of how either of you currently feel about it.

What both of you need is to find ways to blow off steam, activities the two of you can do together or separately to release the tension before it gets the best of you and escalates into all-out verbal warfare, or worse, an extended, silent stalemate. Having the means and the wherewithal to temporarily remove yourselves from the stress of expectant parenthood and enter a peaceful parallel universe is vital to you and your partner's mental health and the well-being of your relationship.

Bottom line: do whatever it takes to purge yourselves of the poisonous stress that often comes with pregnancy and to reconnect with one another when it appears you are drifting apart. Here are a few suggestions for reclaiming your sanity and restoring a sense of calm amid the chaos:

▶ **MAKE A DATE.** Set aside the to-do list and reserve tonight or some night in the not-too-distant future for an outing in which the two of you—and some friends, if you feel like socializing—focus on enjoying one another's company in a relaxed setting. Make a reservation at your favorite restaurant and vow not to dwell on baby-related topics at the dinner table (it tends to bore your childless friends to tears anyway). Take in a movie. Play some darts. Tote your bowling balls to the local lanes to roll a few frames. Take a salsa dancing lesson together.

▶ **LEAVE THE CAVE.** If your skin has a fluorescent sheen, perhaps it's because you have been pent up indoors all week. Make a point of getting out of the house—take a drive in the countryside, go for an extended walk, tend to your livestock or check on the barley and hops crops you have been cultivating to supply your home beer-brewing operation.

▶ **GET SOME EXERCISE.** Few things relieve tension as well as a good sweat and endorphin release. Go for a hike, take a bike ride, go for a swim, hit the gym for a workout, have sex, pound the heavy bag for a while.

▶ **FIND A NEW HOBBY.** You've always wanted to take up knitting, caveman. Maybe now is the time to do so. Have a guitar gathering dust in the closet? Get it tuned, restrung, and ready for you to begin teaching yourself or taking lessons. Been intrigued lately by the prospect of turning part of your basement into a beer-brewing operation so you can craft and stock your own homebrew? Ask some buddies who share your taste in suds if they're interested in partnering in a homebrew operation.

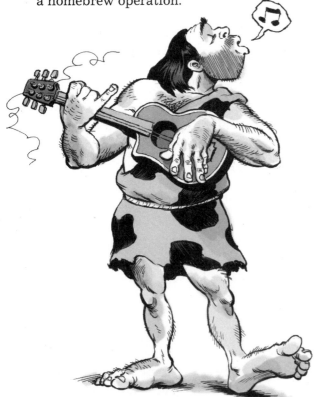

Brewing as a means of meeting the beer-supply needs of your household is one example of how hobbies can be channeled to constructive use. The same goes for knitting, a skill that allows you to produce blankets, hats, mittens, scarves, and other items for the baby. There are other hobbies that bring tangible benefits to the pregnant household. The guy who takes up woodworking can produce rudimentary pieces for the nursery: shelving, a stool, or even a toy box. The caveman who resolves to become a competent chef, as Gronk did when he had a kid on the way, cultivates a lifelong skill that can bring lasting benefits to himself, his woman, the baby, and whomever else happens to be sharing a meal with them. And the expectant father who takes up gardening can supply himself with ingredients—vegetables, fruits, herbs—for the meals he cooks.

▶ **MOVIE DAY.** When the weather is particularly lousy outdoors, rather than let your pregnancy anxieties drive the two of you stir crazy, rent a stack of movies, pop some popcorn, draw the curtains, and settle in for a marathon home-cinema session. Will it be the classic series of *Hellraiser* movies or a few seasons of *Sex and the City*?

▶ **VICE NIGHT.** With the onset of pregnancy began the campaign to purge bad habits and vices in the name of becoming a responsible parent-to-be. But all work and no joy makes Cro-Magnon a dull boy. Here's your chance to backslide on some of those bad habits for one day and *one day only*. Go ahead, caveman, get out the lawn darts, enjoy a cigar, watch football all day.

► **FIND MENIAL, MINDLESS, NONTAX-ING TASKS** that feed the nesting urge and make you feel like you're doing something constructive. Sometimes pending parenthood can paralyze the mind and body. Here's one way to break the inertia.

► **GO YOUR OWN WAY.** Pick a night when the caveman and woman grant one another hall passes to pursue single-sex social activities, known in the beer commercials as "guys night out" and "femme night," only in your case it comes without the writhing dance floor scenes and cheerleaders. Your caveman comrades (none of whom have recently had anything resembling a relationship with a female, it could be pointed out) have long accused you of surrendering your manhood and abandoning them. With guy's night out, you have a chance to reconnect with them, reassert yourself, and prove that your glands are still prolific (though now somewhat more erratic) testosterone producers. Your woman, meanwhile, gets a break from you and a chance to rekindle her own sense of independence. This needn't be a one-shot deal, either. Regularly carving out time for individual pursuits is important for any couple, expectant or otherwise. Doing your own thing helps each of you gain perspective on your situation and an appreciation of one another's contributions to the pregnancy partnership. One night out with your muttonhead buddies, listening to their absurd attempts to engage females in conversation and their inane fantasy football prattle, also provides a valuable reminder that having a solid relationship with a woman and a baby on the way isn't such a bad thing.

► **PAMPER YOURSELVES.** It may not come cheaply, but nothing relieves and cleanses tension like a visit to the spa. For the woman, there's the opportunity to get a prenatal massage, a manicure or a pedicure, a facial, and other popular means of rejuvenating mind, body, and spirit. As for the caveman, who may never have had the pleasure of an extended spa visit, here is his opportunity to explore techniques—such as a hot-stone massage, a mud wrap, and a session in the sweat lodge—that certainly will appeal to his Stone Age sensibilities.

However, contrary to what you've heard in the locker room, there are no "happy endings" to be had here. Your woman is in the room next door, your masseuse is an accredited and ethical massage therapist, and this isn't one of those illegal "massage parlors" where what's on the menu doesn't reflect all the services rendered.

► **TAKE A LONG WEEKEND AWAY.** Pregnancy has cut into your chances to travel as a couple. What you need is a few days away in the mountains, on the beach, or anyplace where relaxation and leisure pursuits are a top priority. Two nights may not suffice. Reward yourself with a long weekend of at least three nights away. Drive, fly, take the train, whatever it takes to leave town. And keep in mind, the earlier you take a weekend away, the less likely your woman is to have pregnancy-related travel restrictions or a lack of energy to keep her at home. One weekend getaway is nice during pregnancy; two is even better; three is optimal but not always feasible from a time or financial standpoint.

▶ **RECONNECT WITH NATURE.** One way to escape town at a low cost—and in a manner that's especially appealing to the caveman—is camping. Spending a night or two sleeping outdoors in unspoiled nature is a great way for the two of you to forget the rat race, recharge your batteries, and enjoy campsite activities that help you reconnect with your primal hunter-gatherer instincts: scavenging firewood, building a fire, eating only what you can catch (or fit in the cooler), and cooking food on a stick.

It's wise to get your camping out of the way earlier in the pregnancy term, since sleeping on a camp mattress on the cold, hard ground holds little appeal for a woman in her third (or even second) trimester. Also, while winter camping and sleeping in a snow cave you fashioned with your own hands is admirable, now is not the time to test your survival skills in that environment. Stick to camping in conditions that make your woman as comfortable as possible and don't begrudge her bringing a hair dryer, a

harem's worth of pillows, and other creature comforts to the campsite. After all, it was you who brought the diesel generator to power the electric tiki torches.

▶ **COMPARE NOTES AND EXPERIENCES WITH OTHERS** in the same state of expectancy as you. If the two of you are taking some kind of prenatal birthing or parenting class, that's an excellent forum for sharing your anxieties, observations, and advice with other "primi" couples and the person teaching the class. Or if you prefer getting advice from peers who have already gone through a pregnancy or two, you probably know a few couples who can provide the guidance and know-how you seek. It may even be worth seeking out advice from your parents, though their memories of pregnancy and childbirth may not be very fresh.

▶ **GO SHOPPING.** Sometimes it just feels good to spend money. So whether you want to scratch a few things off the list of baby items to buy or you merely want to scratch an itch to spend frivolously on luxury items, immersing yourselves in shameless consumer behavior may provide the two of you with the temporary solace you crave.

FROM WOMB TO WALLET: BUDGETING FOR BABY

A flurry of big-ticket baby-gear acquisitions and impulsive purchases leaves the caveman in you yearning for the days when commerce was based largely on barter. "My oxen and I will plow your field before the next planting season in exchange for that crib."

While the barter system has largely gone the way of the oxen cart, there remain plenty of other methods the cagey couple can use to reduce the potentially steep tab they stand to run up in making their home fit for a baby. Since the two of you are not a government entity, you likely don't have a limitless credit line or the wherewithal to unflinchingly amass huge debts. That means that unlike Uncle Sam, you must adhere to some semblance of a budget and maintain at least a shred of fiscal responsibility.

The cost of pregnancy, childbirth, and parental preparation can mount quickly. Items such as a crib, changing table, rocking chair, stroller, and car seat must be procured. Your baby must have a wardrobe ready for his or her hospital stay and return home. The nursery must be decorated and equipped according to the chosen motif; here a caveman likes a pastoral motif featuring an earthen floor, hay bales, stone cairns, and real livestock, while his woman prefers one with softer and more abstract references to animalia and the Paleolithic lifestyle.

PONDER THIS

HOW WELL ARE YOU COVERED?

Gronk was one of the lucky ones. He and his woman had a health insurance policy that covered all but a couple hundred dollars of the $15,000 hospital tab for the birth of their child. Others who aren't so fortunate because their coverage is less extensive or they lack coverage altogether may find themselves footing a major bill for the few days they spend at a birthing facility. Of course, the investment is well worth it. But added up, all those items on a birth-related bill—for things such as the anesthesiologist's time, the cost of a labor-inducing drip, the hourly tab for the OB-GYN during delivery, and of course, the Salisbury steaks you enjoyed for the celebratory postbirth meal—can stretch a budget to the breaking point if you're not prepared. Given how widely coverage varies from insurance carrier to insurance carrier, it's smart to contact your health insurance provider well before the birth to find out exactly what the company will and won't cover. It's also worthwhile to obtain precertification from your carrier that the birthing facility you are planning to use is an approved provider. Rather than sweating about the cost of an extra night's stay in the hospital, a precertified couple can instead reserve their perspiration for the huge task at hand. If you or your partner don't have health insurance or can't afford to get it, state agencies across the country have prenatal care programs that you should take advantage of. Speak to a public health care official for your state and learn about guidelines and opportunities for your family.

Other necessities also come at a cost: medical care for your woman during pregnancy and for both her and the baby after childbirth; any home improvements you can't make yourselves, from building an addition to ridding your home of hazards such as asbestos and radon. If you have a vehicle that lacks space to accommodate a car seat, you need to find one that does. The two of you also may feel compelled to add items you don't need but want for the sake of preserving lifestyle, memories, and/or sanity: baby jogger, video camera, minivan with multiple DVD screens, nursery surveillance system, etc.

Remember, while buying brand new and top-of-the-line is nice, it's not always necessary. Before you rush to get a second job or seriously consider the cash-generating possibilities of a caveman stud service involving you and your buddies, here's a small consolation: play your cards correctly and the two of you should not have to overextend yourselves. Here's why:

- Items such as cribs, changing tables, strollers, and joggers can be readily had for pennies on the dollar at **secondhand stores** (some specializing in things baby-related) and **yard sales**. The quality can be spotty, but usually with persistence and a discerning eye, you can find durable items in a good state of repair with plenty of mileage left. Yard sales also provide the caveman with an ideal opportunity to assert his skills as a haggler. "Says on the sticker you want twenty-five dollars for this collapsible stroller. Usually an item like this retails for seventy-five bucks new. How about if we meet in the middle at fifty dollars?" *Sold!*

- Encourage someone to throw you a **baby shower**. No single baby-related event rivals the baby shower in terms of overall no-cost yield. What's more, the two of you can publicize the existence of your gift registry, where you painstakingly develop a wish list specifying to invitees exactly what items you want and where you want them to purchase it. And further, since etiquette dictates that every person who is invited must furnish a gift, even if they cannot attend, the more folks you invite, the more shower gifts you are apt to receive. For a less well-off couple, this is a strategically shrewd move. The trade-off is that the two of you (or just your woman if—count your blessings—it's a female-only shower) must endure the actual event, including the exceedingly tedious and sometimes awkward gift-opening exercise. If you have advanced through several months of pregnancy without word of a shower being held in your honor, it's time to start planting the seed with subtle hints to potential hosts and hostesses. Your lack of tact and cunning makes this a task better performed by your woman.

- Scout the **Internet** for new and used equipment. Online classified listings and auction sites offer attractive prices on quality, name-brand baby gear.

- Establish a **trading pool** with friends and relatives in which pool members agree to buy clothes and to share them with other members of the pool in a hand-me-down chain. Once a kid grows out of some clothes, they're sent along to other pool members to outfit their children. Meanwhile, when other children of pool members grow out of clothes, if they are not too worn or soiled, they are sent along to other kids or returned to the original user in time to be worn by his or her next offspring.

▶ If the pooling concept seems a bit too commune-like for you, there are plenty of other hand-me-down clothing sources. Look to **friends, relatives, yard sales, and secondhand stores** for "gently worn" clothing. It may not always be stylish and it likely won't look totally new, but style and shine don't matter to a two-month old anyway.

Ask friends and relatives who have exited child-production mode and thus no longer need their baby equipment if they have anything in storage they want to shed. Here's an excellent chance to secure potentially pricey items such as cribs at no charge. Donors may even appreciate you freeing space in their basement by taking unused items off their hands. So as not to make this a one-sided deal, Citizen Caveman, here's a chance to exercise your barter techniques by offering your services—to fertilize the garden, to help reshingle the roof—as a show of goodwill and thanks to the parties who supplied the items.

BOAR IN THE HEADLIGHTS

Yeah, he was blinded by the light
Cut loose like a deuce, another runner
* in the night*
Blinded by the light
He got down but she never got tight, but
* he's gonna make it tonight*

—BRUCE SPRINGSTEEN,
"BLINDED BY THE LIGHT"

The mind is a powerful and mysterious instrument, even when it is housed in the cavernous cranium of a caveman. During particularly stressing or trying times, expectant fatherhood among them, the goings-on inside a contemporary Cro-Magnon's head can manifest themselves in some very odd ways.

During his woman's pregnancy, for example, it's not unusual for a guy to develop physical manifestations that stem from a pervasive feeling of powerlessness, a sense that his fate is in the hands of an invisible—and not necessarily benevolent—force. Oftentimes that sense of impotence will be exacerbated by a feeling that his needs are being overshadowed by those of his pregnant partner.

There's comfort in knowing you are not alone in harboring such feelings. On the next page we've listed some of the issues Gronk confronted during his woman's pregnancy, with their likely cause and the means he found to relieve them.

COMMON CRO-MAGNON CONDITIONS & COPING MECHANISMS

SOURCE OF ANGST	MANIFESTATION	SOURCE OF RELIEF
Fear that child will resemble oneself too much	Losing hair/fur in large clumps	A quick genetics lesson provides comfort that baby will have at least some of mother's features
Extreme stress, overtiredness	An acute case of shingles	Prescription medication, faith the pain will subside
Too much to do, too little time	Episodes of sleepwalking	A weeklong visit from father or father-in-law to help with household projects
Racing thoughts, baseless fears, and legitimate anxieties	Insomnia	An evening cocktail, glass of wine, or bottle of beer
Concerns about safety of expectant mother, fetus/newborn	Nightmares: not the usual ones (showing up to work naked, teeth crumbling in one's mouth), but extremely vivid scenes in which the man's woman and newborn are threatened	Remove weapon collection (clubs, spears, bow and arrows) from storage for sharpening, shining
Feeling neglected, overlooked	Couvade symptoms: backache, nausea, expanding midsection	Extended conversations with guys who have been through pregnancy
Juggling pregnancy, work, relationships	Inertia bordering on clinical depression	Consult friends, relatives, books, and other expert sources for advice, sympathy
Neglect of accustomed male-type outlets	Pacing, fidgeting, attention deficiency	Reconnect with buddies and prehistoric pastimes
Lack of sexual activity	Pubescent dreams, nocturnal emissions, cold showers, excessive exercise	"Imaginary lover—satisfaction guaranteed"
Financial worries	Extreme tightfistedness: three-shower-per-week limit to cut water bill; thermostat set at 50°F during the dead of winter; ramen noodles in regular meal rotation	Put together a household budget/ spending plan

HEEDING THE CALL OF THE INNER CAVEMAN

Something about a caveman attracts certain modern women, even ones considered highly cultured, and it almost certainly isn't his polish, his social graces, or the company he keeps. More likely it is an animal attraction in which the female is drawn to him because of such things as his scent and because of the clumps of hair that poke from the edges of his clothing, plus his clumsy attempts to pass as a modern man.

Your woman chose you perhaps because her tastes tend toward the primitive, so there's no sense in trying to bury the caveman inside you. Sometimes you must honor and obey your true self. Your willingness to evolve into a true partner during pregnancy and parenthood at least earns you the right to occasionally pursue the prehistoric pastimes you have always enjoyed. Some of those pursuits are done as a couple and some the caveman does *sans* woman. If you keep a healthy balance between the two, you will have activities that strengthen your bond and preserve your passion as an expectant couple on the one hand, and on the other, you

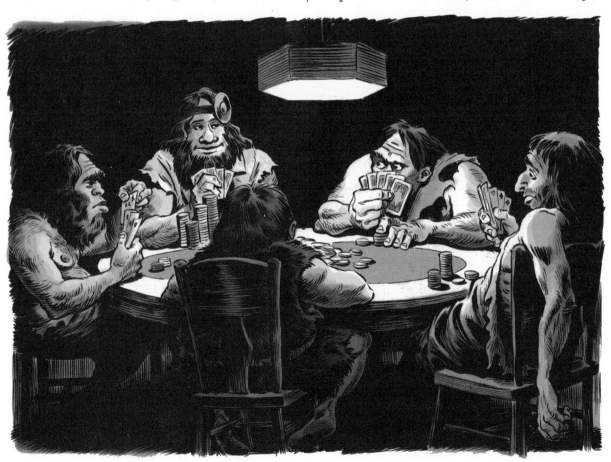

will have activities that each of you do independently, either with friends or alone.

Being a partner in pregnancy is about sharing the load and compromising, but for both of you, it is about being true to yourself. Staying happy (or at least sane) means not denying one another and yourself the things you enjoy and crave most, because if you feel you're sacrificing too much during pregnancy, you're apt to become resentful or feel as if you're losing your identity. And no one wants to be around a sullen, emotionally wounded caveman.

Below are some suggested activities for the expectant father to undertake in order to stay true to his inner caveman:

	SINGLE	DUO
Try new things to keep from getting stuck in your ways	X	X
Play poker with friends, usually a guys-only activity; resist the urge to overdo it with too many poker nights	X	
Massage/spa treatments, including primal stone massage, mud wrap, and Turkish rub	X	X
Stay active with sports/activities such as softball, volleyball, hoops, hiking, biking, weightlifting, dance	X	X
Fantasy football, rotisserie baseball, and other stats-based excuses for small-time wagering	X	
A weekend away, either as a guys-only trip (your woman has no desire to be there), as a couple, or with the two of you and perhaps some friends, as well	X	X
Hunting, fishing, other excuses to wear camouflage, stalk prey, fire weapons	X	

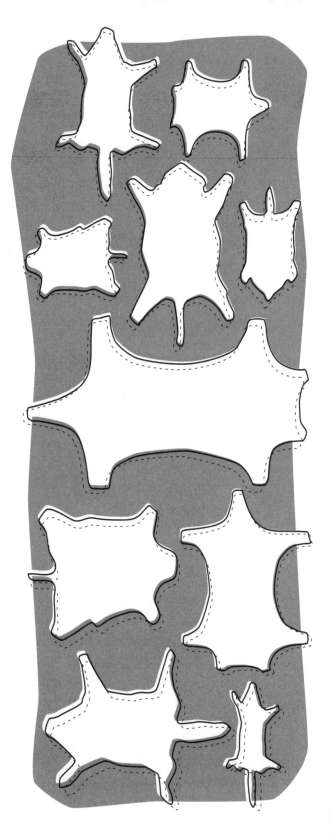

CHAPTER 3

THE CAN-DO CAVEMAN (A.K.A. HOMO HABILIS)

You're as helpless as a baby
But I love you, understand
I'm just gettin' tired
Of being your ole handy man
Your woman's getting tired of being
*   your ole handy man*

—DOLLY PARTON, "YOUR OLE HANDY MAN"

NOW IS A good time to pause for a moment and reflect on a past chapter of your caveman life—your days as a bachelor, when life was simple and the only person for whom you had responsibility was you. You came and went as you pleased, ate what you wanted when you wanted, washed and groomed often enough not to offend, and dated whoever showed interest.

Even during those footloose, fancy-free days you remember so fondly, the burden of taking care of yourself could sometimes be too much for a knuckledragger like you to bear. Recall, for example, how you retreated to your parents' home on a weekly basis to

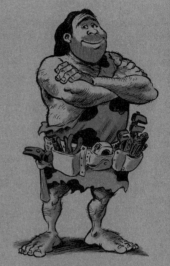

GROW WITH GRONK

What the caveman stands to gain from reading Chapter 3:

▶ **AN UNDERSTANDING** of the next life stage he is entering and the personal evolution he is about to undertake as an expectant father

▶ **A GRASP** of which habits he should keep during pregnancy and which he should drop

▶ **THE SKILLS** to put his hands to good use during pregnancy as his woman's personal prenatal massage slave

▶ **STRATEGIES** for preparing the home, yard, and pet for baby's arrival

▶ **FAMILIARITY** with the various pieces of equipment he will be expected to lug home and assemble

▶ **INSIGHT** into what it takes to turn a room into a baby nursery

▶ **THE KNOW-HOW** to perform CPR on an infant

get your laundry done, cop a rare home-cooked meal, and escape the maelstrom of maleness that was your apartment.

Things started to change when you got serious with a woman. For the first time since you left the cave of your kin and set out on your own, you had to answer to someone other than yourself. Suddenly a person outside your close-knit crew of caveman friends (and a female no less!) desired your attention and companionship—and you were more than happy to oblige. Here at last was someone of the opposite sex who wanted to connect with the true inner caveman lurking behind the protruding brow and excessive body hair. It took some adjusting, but you were cool with the relationship dynamic. The perks of having a steady woman outweighed the flak you caught from your buddies for compromising your caveman values and lifestyle.

But as you eventually came to find, compromise is a necessary ingredient to sustaining a relationship with a woman. That became abundantly clear to you when you took the next step and moved in with a female or actually married one. This uniting of households is where the me-first caveman officially resigned himself to the greater good of the we-first couple. This time, the adjustment came more painfully because it entailed truly sharing your life and personal space with someone you called "wife," "lover," "babe," "cookie," "hon," or just plain "woman."

Now, with a baby on the way, the evolution continues. The next phase of life is about to throw some major challenges your way, so it's time to set aside your sentimentality about those carefree days of yore to prepare for another big dose of reality. The me-first chapter of your life is closed. Now begins the she-first chapter, to be followed roughly nine months later by the wee-one-first chapter.

Self-improvement is essential to meeting the mental and physical challenges that loom as an expectant father. With the well-being of your woman and baby at stake, the situation demands that you shape yourself into a responsible, well-equipped parent-to-be. Here's your chance to become a man among cavemen, to better yourself to the benefit of those who must share the cave with you. Since you are so open to expanding your horizons as a man—and you really have no choice but to be open—we have written a chapter specifically with your personal betterment in mind.

Your mission: to become a modern-day *Homo habilis*. "Handy man" in Latin, *Homo habilis* is thought to be the first direct ancestor of mankind to make and use primitive tools. If some of our earliest descendants could use tools 2.6 million years ago with their limited mental capacity, there's no excuse for you not to use them today.

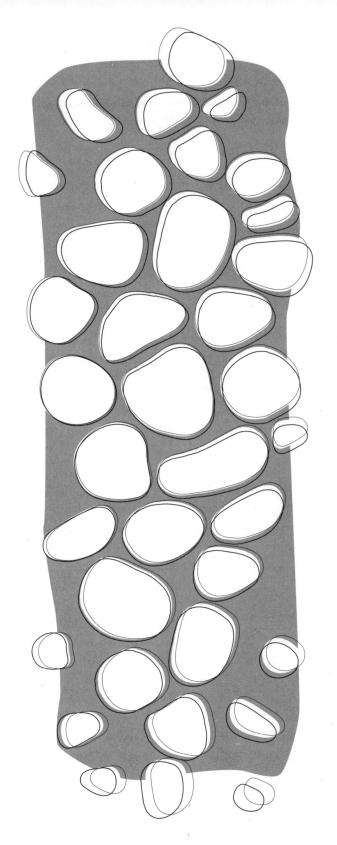

DR. JEKYLL & MR. GRONK

They say old habits die hard. That's especially true for contemporary Cro-Magnons, whose limited worldview renders them true creatures of habit. Oftentimes it takes a jarring event such as pregnancy to knock them out of their comfort zone and force them to take a long, hard look at the man staring

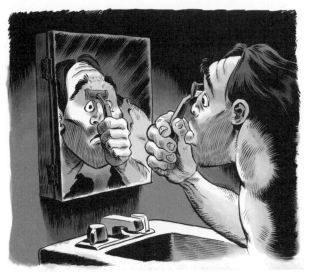

back at them in the mirror. Granted, there's not much a caveman can do about his apish gait or lack of rhythm on the dance floor. In other facets of life, however, he holds his destiny in his own hairy palms. He can and *must* recognize and address his shortcomings, dropping habits that are inappropriate to carry into expectant fatherhood while adopting (or perpetuating) those that make him a more constructive, less obstructive member of the pregnant household. Check out the suggestions on the following chart.

DROP/STOP

THE TOBACCO HABIT. The smokes and/or chew must go. Smoking, chewing, and their byproducts, secondhand smoke and tobacco juice, are health hazards for you, mom-to-be, and womb-bound baby.

HOSTING UNANNOUNCED, MARATHON POKER GAMES. Move the party to a bachelor friend's where there's always beer in the fridge and never a woman to disturb.

USING FOUL LANGUAGE. Substitute unintelligible grunts for cussing. It's just as satisfying.

THE EXPECTATION THAT DINNERS WILL BE PREPARED FOR YOU: The onus is now on you to at least share cooking duties, big fella.

RECKLESS (and especially in the caveman's case, potentially life-threatening) **ACTIVITIES.** ATV racing, fencing, crossbow hunting, base-jumping; no-pads tackle football

GAMBLING: What used to be disposable income is now your future child's college fund.

SNORING. Pregnant women value their sleep above almost anything, so do whatever it takes to keep your nocturnal noises from disturbing her—wear a Breathe-Rite, trim your nose hair, remove the cat from your face.

COMMUNICATING WITH OLD FLAMES. You couldn't pick a worse time to reconnect with an "ex." If your senior prom date sends you an unsolicited e-mail, go ahead and respond. But the repartee stops there; no online chatting or text-messaging.

STAYING OUT LATE WITHOUT CHECKING IN. Your woman needs to know the father of her child is safe. Don't leave her hanging, lest your evening hall-pass privileges be revoked.

QUASH THE COLOGNE. The pungent, "liquid love" pheromone potion your woman once tolerated (because it masked other, more offensive odors) is now downright nauseating to her.

DEVELOP/KEEP

HANDYMAN SKILLS. The ability to tackle household projects with manual and/or power tools, always taking care to protect digits

INSTEAD OF WATCHING THE GAME ON TV, couchbound, listen to it on the radio while you do something constructive.

A TASTE FOR HOUSEHOLD CHORES. Take on the dishes, the laundry, vacuuming, feeding the dog, cleaning out the cat box.

IMPROVED CLEANLINESS AND GROOMING HABITS. Discard decade-old canvas sneakers inhabited by centipedes; clip nose hair and nails regularly; learn to hit the bowl, not the seat, when urinating.

CAN-DO IN THE KITCHEN. The ability to cook delicious, nutritious meals that don't come in a can, box, or microwaveable container

GROCERY SHOPPING AND OTHER HUNTING AND GATHERING ERRANDS, often at a moment's notice

A SILVER TONGUE that's always ready with compliments and positive comments for your lady: "When it comes to women's underwear, honey, I love the big stuff."

A VOLUNTEER MENTALITY. Offer to open doors, carry heavy items, do chores, give massages.

TUNE IN, TAKE NOTE. You're no mind reader, so when your woman is engaging you in conversation, use those oversize flaps attached to your head to absorb, not deflect, what she's saying.

KEEP UP THE GOOD WORK. Stick with the chores you already perform, such as cutting the grass, taking out the trash, watering the plants, etc.

A WILLINGNESS TO SLEEP IN THE GUEST ROOM OR ON THE COUCH, UPON REQUEST. A queen-size bed can seem small with a pregnant woman in there with you, especially during the third trimester, when she's at her largest and her sleep can be especially fitful.

IN UTERO, IN STEREO

Anyone who has mixed it up in a mosh pit, heard Pink Floyd's *The Wall* on headphones, or gently swayed to a power ballad can attest to music's ability to soothe, to excite, to stimulate. And just as some classic, bone-crunching Led Zeppelin can send tingles down a caveman's spine, so too can a fetus respond to the sounds and rhythms it hears *in utero*. Indeed, some medical research shows that the music a fetus hears in the womb may encourage development of the fetal brain. Something else to consider: while you will never be mistaken for a young Michael Jackson (or, heaven forbid, a middle-aged M.J.) on the dance floor, by introducing a little music to your baby while still in the womb, he or she may enter the world with the sense of rhythm you clearly lack.

Flip on the surround sound, have your woman position her belly within earshot of the speakers, and let the music flow. Here

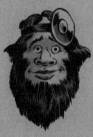

DR. BRIAN

BORN WITH A BLACK LUNG: THE EVILS OF SECONDHAND SMOKE

....

Do you mind if I smoke?
No, do you mind if I fart?

—STEVE MARTIN

....

Among all the bad habits an expectant father can bring into a pregnancy, smoking is among the worst because of the effects secondhand smoke can have on a pregnant woman, the developing baby, and others around you. Secondhand smoke causes or exacerbates a range of adverse health effects, from cancer to respiratory infections, and is named as the cause for about 3,000 lung cancer deaths and 35,000 heart disease deaths annually among adult non-smokers in the United States. Research shows that nonsmokers who are exposed to secondhand smoke are 25 percent more likely to have coronary heart diseases compared to nonsmokers not exposed to smoke.

Secondhand smoke doesn't just harm adults. In fact, its effects can reach into the womb. For example, a recent study found that secondhand cigarette smoke can cause genetic mutations in a fetus that can lead to leukemia and lymphoma. Secondhand smoke is named as the culprit for 150,000 to 300,000 lower respiratory tract infections in infants and children less than eighteen months of age, resulting in between 7,500 and 15,000 hospitalizations each year in the United States. Here is another even more shocking statistic: secondhand smoke causes an estimated 1,900 to 2,700 sudden infant death syndrome (SIDS) deaths in the nation annually.[1] Need we say more about the imperative to quit?

If these figures don't convince you of the evils of secondhand (and firsthand) smoke, check out ALA's Tobacco Morbidity and Mortality Trend Report or its Lung Disease Data publication in the Data and Statistics section of the organization's website, lungusa.org, or call 800-LUNG-USA.

---

1. American Lung Association. Secondhand Smoke Fact Sheet. http://www.lungusa.org/site/pp.asp?c=dvLUK9O0E&b=35422 (accessed Oct. 24, 2005).

are some relevant selections for the prenatal jukebox and perhaps for a mix tape/CD/iPod playlist you make to play in the delivery room:

- "Baby We've Got a Date" by Bob Marley (a classic reggae song to remind the baby to stick to the due date he or she was assigned by the doctor)
- "Sweet Child of Mine" by Guns N' Roses
- "I Got You Babe" (the UB40/Chrissie Hynde version preferred over Sonny & Cher)
- "Stay Up Late" by Talking Heads
- "My Baby Don't Tolerate" by Lyle Lovett
- "Love to Love You Baby" by Donna Summer
- "Baby I Love Your Way" by Peter Frampton
- "Ooo Baby Baby" by Smokey Robinson & the Miracles
- "It's All Over Now Baby Blue" by Bob Dylan
- Anything off *Learning to Crawl* by the Pretenders
- "Is You Is or Is You Ain't My Baby" by Dinah Washington (a question to pose when there's a mix-up in the hospital nursery)
- "Wild Child" by Lou Reed
- Any animal-related or silly song by the Beatles, "Piggies," "Rocky Raccoon," "Blackbird," "Octopus's Garden," "Yellow Submarine" among them
- "Voodoo Chile" by Jimi Hendrix

RUB THE ONE YOU'RE WITH: PRENATAL MASSAGE FOR KNUCKLEDRAGGERS

Vincent: Have you ever given a foot massage?
Jules: [scoffs] Don't be tellin' me about foot massages. I'm the foot %@#!& master.*
Vincent: Given a lot of 'em?
Jules: $@#& yeah. I got my technique down and everything. I don't be ticklin' or nothin'.

—PULP FICTION

One of the great unknowns of pregnancy, at least from the male perspective, is how childbearing will affect a woman's sexual urges. Every woman responds differently; some respond unpredictably. For example, one who is frisky at various points in the gestation period could at other times seem downright disinterested (the word *frigid* should not be part of your vocabulary unless you are speaking of the temperature outdoors). It is during those dry spells that the caveman may feel a case of benign neglect, his primal need for intimacy unfulfilled.

Even when sexual activity isn't an option—and sometimes an overwhelmed caveman can be the cause for curbed sexual activity, a phenomenon we'll investigate in Chapter 5—it is crucial for both of you to maintain a sense of physical intimacy, lest you lose the physical connection that is vital to many relationships. Here's where the ancient art of massage can do wonders, helping the expectant couple recapture some of the intimacy that may be lost, at least temporarily, during the childbearing months. Applied properly, when the time is right (hormonal and planetary alignment), with just the right amount of oil, the massage techniques you learn may prove to be a powerful seduction tool even a weary pregnant woman cannot resist.

But let's not lose sight of why prenatal massage exists in the first place: to benefit the pregnant mom before and during labor. By learning and applying a few simple techniques, the expectant father can use his touch to bring his woman comfort and relief from the aches and pains that often come with her expanding dimensions, added weight, and shifting center of gravity.

Your hands are strong from years of brandishing heavy clubs, moving boulders out of your path, and hauling heavy items (logs, animal carcasses, etc.) back to the cave. During pregnancy, those hands should be busy most of the time (and hopefully not just on your own body parts). Massage allows you to put your hands to constructive use. Not only do the techniques you're about to learn come in handy during pregnancy, you also can employ them during labor to relax your partner and help relieve discomfort and cramps.

Prenatal massage puts the power to help a woman and the developing baby squarely in the caveman's hairy hands. Beyond relieving pain or discomfort in areas such as the back, shoulders, neck, feet, calves, pelvis, and hips, massage offers a wide range of other benefits:

- It improves the flow of nourishment to the baby by increasing the mom's circulation.

- It stabilizes hormone levels by stimulating glandular secretions, which can help level some of the emotional and physical peaks and valleys of pregnancy.

- It improves digestion, perhaps alleviating common symptoms such as heartburn.

- It reduces fatigue and swelling.

- It improves the skin's elasticity, reducing the chance of pregnancy-related stretch marks appearing.

- It supports gestation by encouraging cellular regeneration while helping carry away lactic acid and cellular waste that can cause muscle fatigue.

- It relieves stress and tension, providing relaxation that can lead to an easier birth and quicker postpartum recovery.

- It can help the expectant mom sleep better, with less discomfort.

WHEN MASSAGE MIGHT NOT BE APPROPRIATE (CONTRAINDICATIONS)

You and your woman are anxious to get your home-massage regimen started. But wait. You first need to be aware of certain health issues that suggest a pregnant woman should avoid massage. Use common sense: do not massage your woman if she has been vomiting, has a fever, bloody discharge, or diarrhea. Do not perform massage if she has a malignant condition (cancer). If she has high blood pressure or preeclampsia, a disorder in pregnant women that causes high blood pressure, be sure she gets clearance from her doctor before you let your fingers do the talking. Also, avoid massaging areas where she has varicose veins or skin irritations.

PREPARATION

Before you begin practicing as an amateur masseur, you need to get your hands in proper massage condition so the grip you apply is supple, not rough and clumsy. That means cutting your fingernails so they won't scratch the massage subject. Also consider using a pumice stone over the course of a few days to slough the calluses from your hands. The pumice stone also is a good grooming tool to use on feet—your woman's and your own. Shaving your hairy palms is also a wise move. While having baby-soft hands may afford you less protection in your tree-climbing and vine-swinging pursuits, your woman will appreciate being massaged by a well-manicured man.

Before you start rubbing, also be sure your hands are warm and clean. The massage won't last thirty seconds if your mitts are icy and gritty.

TOOLS OF THE TRADE

The well-prepared caveman masseur also has to get the right massage tools, many of which he may already have in-house. Here are some items you will need:

▶ **CANDLES** (mildly scented or unscented)

▶ **PILLOWS** for support (a special "body" pillow works well, particularly when she's being massaged while lying on her side)

▶ **TOWELS**

▶ **MUSIC** that's soothing, not too loud or intrusive, so as not to hinder conversation and concentration. Some couples find the massage experience is more intimate without music.

▶ **MASSAGE OIL** (see Desirae's Prenatal Massage Potion on p. 43)

THE SETTING

You want your woman to relax and be comfortable during and after the massage, so pick a quiet place to work your magic. Turn off telephones and the television set, dim the lights (but not so much you can't see your subject), and light some candles to create the right mood.

Since most households lack a massage table, you will need to find a surface on which your massage "client" can sit or lie comfortably while you get busy on her body. The bed is a good place (especially when massage turns into foreplay), as is a couch, a cozy chair, or a recliner. A foot massage works well when your woman is in the bathtub.

AREAS OF THE BODY TO FOCUS ATTENTION

It's not uncommon for a pregnant woman to report that she "hurts all over." The caveman's first instinct as a novice masseur is to narrow his focus to the areas of her body

DESIRAE'S PRENATAL MASSAGE POTION

Professional massage therapists, including certified prenatal massage specialist Desirae, a member of the Expectant Caveman's Ad Hoc Female Advisory Council, prefer oil over lotion because its gliding qualities last longer on the surface of the skin. Amateur masseurs can prepare their own massage oil by following Desirae's home recipe:

2 TEASPOONS base oil: castor, jojoba, soybean or extra virgin olive oil

3 DROPS "spike" lavender essential oil ("spike" should be indicated on the label)

I DROP chamomile essential oil

I DROP geranium essential oil

The amounts of each ingredient provide enough for one massage session. By properly multiplying each measurement, you can mix a larger batch to last multiple sessions. Your local natural foods store should stock any of the items you don't already have on hand. While the ingredients in Desirae's potion are pretty mild, your woman's nose may not agree with olive oil, for example, in which case you can use one of the other base oils.

he finds most intriguing. But at least for the moment, those areas are off limits to his groping hands.

For now, Dr. Digits, you want to focus your efforts on the parts of her body that typically need the most attention because they often bear the brunt of her added weight and shifting proportions—her feet, ankles and calves, her lower back and gluteus (but-

tocks) muscles, and her neck and shoulders. These are the places where your hands can provide the most immediate relief for her aches and pains.

TECHNIQUES

In prehistoric times, a properly administered massage was known as "giving good hand." By practicing the techniques illustrated below, your woman will grow dependent on your skilled hands, to the point where you make massage a regular part of your routine, practiced several times a week or even on a daily basis.

A person who "gives good hand" is one who:

▶ Pays attention to detail in creating a soothing, distraction-free massage environment

▶ Is firm but never rough with his touch

▶ Uses a variety of touching techniques—kneading, rubbing, circular motions, and pressing with fingers, palms, and full hands, applying varying pressures

▶ Focuses on muscles, not bones

▶ Engages the subject in conversation with a soothing voice and honors her wishes when she wants silence

▶ Asks the subject if the pressure he's applying is too little or too much

▶ Takes care not to deliver massage too vigorously or forcefully

▶ Never lets his hands wander unless the subject permits it

▶ Massages evenly and thoroughly

Among the dozens of different "schools" of massage, the Swedish technique is by far the most popular kind practiced in the United States. The Swedish massage school teaches five basic strokes, each of which can be used in prenatal massage:

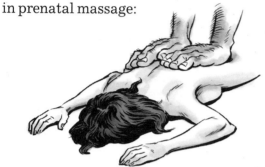

I. EFFLEURAGE: This maneuver, performed with the whole hand or the thumb, incorporates long, gliding strokes, such as along the length of the spine from the neck to the lower back. It allows the masseur to familiarize himself with his subject's body and vice versa.

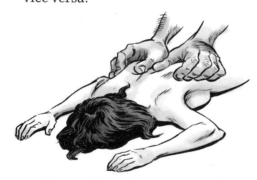

2. PETRISSAGE: A gentle grabbing and lifting of muscles away from the bone, followed by light rolling, pressing, and squeezing to encourage deeper circulation.

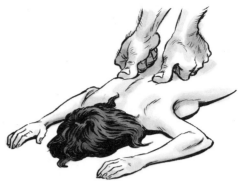

3. FRICTION: Moving the thumbs and fingertips in circular motions to penetrate and deeply work muscles. Great for areas where she feels muscle knots.

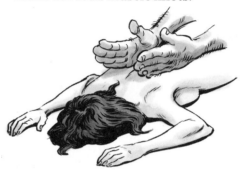

4. TAPOTEMENT: A series of tapping motions applied with the edge of the hand, fingertips, or closed hand, which, if performed properly, helps release tension and muscle cramps.

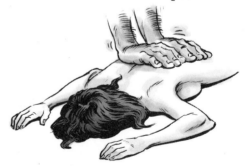

5. VIBRATION: Commonly used to relieve lower back pain. With this technique, the masseur firmly presses and flattens his fingers on a muscle, then shakes the area for a few seconds.

Whether you set aside a full hour to work her over or just ten minutes to relieve her stress, tension, and discomfort, the time you invest will pay huge dividends to both of you. And the best thing about massage is that it's a gift that keeps on giving long after pregnancy. Here's a skill you can use time and again throughout your lifetime to keep family and friends relaxed and comfortable. People who experience your digital prowess firsthand may themselves want to learn some of your techniques for use on others. Now, let's get down to business so you can start spreading the love.

FOOT, ANKLE, AND CALF

WARM-UP Fill a bowl or other container with warm water for her to soak her feet prior to massage. Or draw a bath and, before she gets in, sprinkle rose petals on the surface of the water. This sets a relaxing tone to carry through to the massage. A word of caution when you're incorporating water into your foot massage. Be sure her feet don't get chilled; having cold feet can constrict blood flow to the uterus. So make every effort to keep her feet warm after they've been in water by wrapping them in towels or having socks or slippers ready for her to slip on before you start massaging.

POSITIONING There are several positions in which to receive a foot massage:

1. Lying in the bath, feet and ankles poking out of the water.

2. Lying on the bed, feet just off the edge, in a semireclined position with her upper body propped up by pillows (lying down for too long can constrict blood flow, making her and the baby uncomfortable).

3. Seated in a comfortable chair or recliner where the masseur has access to foot, ankle, and calf.

TECHNIQUES Start with gentle rubbing motions around the belly to connect with mom and the baby. This helps relax everyone involved. Then shift your attention to the foot and lower leg.

Stroke the top of the foot using long, slow rubbing motions with both hands. Be firm with your thumbs. Gradually slide your hands the length of the foot, from the toes to the ankle. Now focus on the bottom of the foot. Use firm fingers and knuckles to make circular motions, then slide firm fingers up and down the arch of the foot. Now gently and slowly pull her toes, squeezing them firmly but not painfully.

Next it's on to the ankle. Rotate the ankle by gently grasping the foot in your hands and moving it in a circular motion. Use fingers to work the area in a gentle manner, avoiding deep pressure around the bones on the inside and the outside of the ankle.

Now the calf: use fingers to pull and spread the muscles there, taking care not to cause her discomfort.

BEWARE According to massage therapists, there are pressure points in the ankle area related to the uterus and vagina that, if pressed hard enough and long enough, can send a woman into premature labor. Your goal is to bring lasting pleasure, relaxation, and relief, not early contractions, so tread lightly in the area.

LOWER BACK AND GLUTES

WARM-UP Draw a bath, sprinkle some rose petals, and let her soak awhile, until she's feeling relaxed and ready. Make sure your hands are warm. Then introduce yourself to the area by putting several drops of oil into your hands and in a few sweeping motions spreading it over the lower back and buttocks area.

POSITIONING Have her sit in a comfortable chair, her back to you. Or have her lay on her side on a bed or couch. A note to the caveman masseur: the bed may be your woman's preferred place to receive a massage. That's fine for her, but you may find it to be somewhat uncomfortable. Here's a good time to remind yourself that the discomfort you're experiencing can't hold a candle to what she must endure during pregnancy and childbirth.

TECHNIQUES After warm-up, use your thumbs to massage the area where her hips meet her spine. Rather than wasting time groping for the right spot, look for dimples in the area, one on each side of the spine. The area to target for massage is about three inches up and three inches out from those dimples.

If you cannot spot any dimples, target the area above the hipbones, taking care not to press too hard on bony structures. Now, in the soft area around the lower back, press and release on the tissue using your knuckle or thumb. To help release tension in the area, hold for three seconds, then release.

Now your roving hands can move lower, to the butt cheeks. Staying close to the sacrum (the part of the vertebra that connects with the pelvis) area, massage in circular motions. Using your thumbs or fingertips, start with little circles and gradually enlarge the area they cover until you are working the entire butt cheek, including the area close to the hip joint. Massage around the ball and socket area, even to the front of the thigh, taking care to work deliberately since the subject may be ticklish in the area.

Hold pressure points on the areas of the buttocks she identifies as tender for three seconds, then release and move on to another pressure point.

If you are massaging your woman while she is lying on her side, do your buttocks work one cheek at a time. In this area of the body, it can be especially handy (given the size of the muscle) to use both hands to massage, with your fingers gripping her hips while your thumbs are massaging around the sacrum and deep into the tissue of the buttocks. Here's where your strong caveman hands and long digits really come in handy.

SHOULDERS, NECK, AND HEAD

WARM-UP Again, why not go with the bath and rose-petal combination? The massage can begin once she's relaxed after a good soak and once your hands are warm. Put several drops of oil into your hands and in a few sweeping motions spread it over the neck, shoulders, and mid-back, warming the tissue with gentle squeezing and kneading. This is your introduction.

POSITIONING Have her sit backward in a comfortable chair, her back to you. Or have her lie on her side on a bed or couch.

TECHNIQUES Use your thumb to apply pressure from the spine out across the tops of the shoulders. Also work from spine to shoulder blades, being sure always to work from the spine outward, not inward toward the spine. If she is lying on her side, work one side, then have her rotate 180 degrees to her other side so you can work the other one.

Move to the spots where she seems tightest to your touch or where she indicates she needs special attention. Using the fleshy part of your thumbs, begin to work in small circles in the areas that need help, adjusting the pressure you apply according to your subject's direction.

Expect to find tender spots along the tops of the shoulders and tucked down near the collarbone. Get in there with the fleshy part of your fingers, working in small, circular motions to help ease these areas.

Now, start massaging the neck area, using your fingertips to gently massage the sides of the neck and the lower head, behind the ears, and on the side of the head. Use your thumbs on the back of her neck and along the outside of the upper spine. With the subject's aid, identify tender points and massage them in a *slow* circular motion.

If your woman wants you to spend time on the head, massage it lightly with your fingertips working around her ears, the sides, and top of her head.

Finally, use your thumbs as pressure points. Have your woman tilt her head back slightly onto your thumbs, creating counter-pressure on an area called the low occipital, where the neck and head meet. Avoid rubbing over the spine and massaging the bones directly.

POST-MASSAGE

If she's up for it, try heat—not that which is generated by your body but from a homemade or store-bought heating pack. You can make one at home with a tube sock you fill with rice and tie off at the open end. Once the massage is over, place the rice-filled sock in the microwave on high for two to three minutes, then, after you verify the sock isn't so hot it will scald your woman out of her state of bliss, have her place it over her neck or on her lower back for five to ten minutes. If you are targeting a larger area with the heat treatment, use a flannel pillowcase instead of a sock; fill it halfway, tie off the open end, and place it in the microwave for four to eight minutes (approximately). Test the temperature of the sack before application.

GO TO A PRO However skilled you become at massage, there likely will be times when the expectant mom wants to put herself in the more experienced hands of an expert. Thus, it's worthwhile to supplement your home-massage routine with visits to a massage therapist whose specialized training in treating pregnant women makes him or her especially skilled at delivering full-body treatments. Consider looking for someone who is a certified "prenatal massage therapist." While massage therapists who lack that certification can still perform massage on an expectant mom, they may not be as well equipped to address her specific pregnancy-related needs, nor as familiar with the techniques to use and avoid on a pregnant woman.

SAFE AT HOME

Our house is a very, very fine house
With two cats in the yard
Life used to be so hard
Now everything is easy
'Cause of you

—CROSBY, STILLS, NASH & YOUNG,
"OUR HOUSE"

The procrastinator in you says, "Why worry?" because your child's projected delivery date is still months away. If you're anything like Gronk, however, you will need every minute of every day during the gestation period to prepare yourself for the birth and all those new parental responsibilities that follow. Preparation doesn't just mean putting yourself in the proper mindset, it entails readying your dwelling, your yard, your vehicle(s), and your pet(s) for the new arrival. Keep in mind that while infants enter this world as cuddly but virtually immobile little burping, gurgling, farting, drooling, pooping, crying machines, as they grow so, too, will their ability to get to items you may never have imagined they could reach.

It's never too early to start prepping. You may even find that performing these kinds of mindless tasks is a good way to burn off nervous energy as you wait for the big day to arrive.

INDOORS

It will be at least six months after your baby is born before he or she begins to crawl and a few months after that before the child begins to walk. But that doesn't mean you shouldn't take steps to make your cave a safer place for baby. Here are a few things to address prior to bringing home the infant:

- Lock away your collection of spears, clubs, arrows, and other hunting/self-defense implements.

- Reposition planters, picture frames, fireplace pokers, and other potential projectiles so they can't fall or tip over and harm a helpless newborn.

- Put anything with poisonous or potentially hazardous ingredients—household cleaning supplies, plants, medicine, etc.—out of harm's way.

- Get your home's heating and cooling ducts and vents cleaned.

- Put away dangling electrical cords and other items that could trip you or mom when carrying the baby.

- Check and test for radon, asbestos, lead paint, and other potential health hazards. With a baby on the way, out of sight is no longer out of mind.

- Cover or reupholster any furniture you want protected from regurgitation, sticky hands, and smeared food (your woman may already have done this in advance of you moving in).

OUTDOORS

Although it will be awhile before your little caveperson ventures unaccompanied outdoors, you still need to stay one step ahead. Take stock of potential outdoor hazards no matter how small:

- Keep common items with hazardous ingredients like antifreeze out of harm's way.
- Keep shovels, hedge clippers, weed whackers, chainsaws, lawn darts, and other sharp or potentially dangerous outdoor implements safely stowed away.
- Cover the hot tub with a childproof cover; put in the pool fence, now.
- Fill any fire pits, ditches, crevasses, etc.
- Remove barbed wire.

THE VEHICLE

Buy and install an infant car seat before your baby is born. With all their bells and whistles, some of these newfangled seats can be fairly complex for the common, uninitiated Cro-Magnon to figure out. To make sure you installed it correctly, drive over to your local fire department and ask someone there to check it. In many areas, firefighters are trained to do just that. If not, they may be able to refer you to someone who is.

Prior to pregnancy, you probably didn't worry much about stocking your vehicle with an emergency kit. Now you should. Keep jumper cables, a flashlight, a blanket, flares, matches or a lighter, and a spare tire and jack (or tire inflation kit) in the vehicle at all times. Emergency food rations are probably unnecessary, contrary to what your survivalist friends insist.

And one final thing: get automobile insurance if you don't have it already.

THE ANIMAL

If fish, birds, lizards, ferrets, gerbils, hamsters, rabbits, or bugs are the only pets in your household, you won't have to worry much about preparing such critters for the arrival of a new baby. But if a dog or a cat is an integral part of your household, you probably have a pet that needs the help of his human companions to make the big adjustment that lies ahead.

With their place in the pecking order potentially threatened, dogs and cats also face potentially stressful life changes during and after pregnancy: less sleep and/or new sleep patterns, a new or inconsistent schedule of walks and exercise, and less human attention. Indeed, if your dog or cat could speak, it would probably tell you it's not too thrilled about the prospect of sharing your home—its turf—with the new arrival. That's especially true with canines, which typically need more human interaction than do felines.

The goal is to get your pet to associate the new baby with positive things, not punishment, being ignored, or upsetting changes in routine. Here are some tips to help your pet make a smooth transition:

- **START PREPARING NOW.** The day the baby comes home is not the time to make changes to your pet's life. Early in the pregnancy, brush up on your dog's obedience skills. If you need to move your cat's litter box, do it gradually—a few feet every week. And if you need to change the spot where the dog or cat sleeps, do so now.

▶ **TAKE YOUR PET TO THE VETERI-NARIAN** to confirm it's in good health and its vaccinations are current.

▶ **TIME FOR A PEDICURE.** Trim your pet's nails (or have a groomer do it) to prevent scratches.

▶ **FOSTER FAMILIARITY.** Allow your pet to smell baby clothes, toys, and baby-related items such as the stroller as you bring them home.

▶ **CURB ENTHUSIASM** for behaviors like jumping, nibbling, and roughhousing so they won't endanger the baby once he or she arrives home. Redirect the pet's energies to toys and the like.

▶ **APPEAL TO THE NOSE.** After the baby's birth, bring the new arrival's blanket or an article of his or her clothing home from the hospital and let your pet smell it. Praise the animal around this new smell. Then, when baby arrives home for the first time, let your pet investigate the newcomer. Often a sniff is all it needs to accept the baby as part of the family. Heap praise on the animal for positive interactions with the infant.

▶ **SPEND QUALITY TIME WITH YOUR PET.** Show the dog or cat you still love it, even though it's lost its place in the pecking order. Set aside time to focus only on your pet, and take the dog with you on walks with the baby.

DR. BRIAN

PREGNANT WOMEN AND TOXOPLASMOSIS

The disease called toxoplasmosis was probably more of a concern for our cave-dwelling forebears than it is for mankind here in the twenty-first century. Sometimes contracted through contact with feline feces or—as many of our mono-browed ancestors learned the hard way when dining around the fire pit—by eating undercooked meat, toxoplasmosis today is a very rare disease. Still, it is one expectant moms and their mates should be wary of and cautious about. There's usually no need for pregnant women to avoid cats altogether. But have your woman talk to her family doctor or OB-GYN about the simple precautions she can take to avoid the disease. One way she can do so is to leave gardening and litter-box duties to you instead of exposing herself to places where cat feces may be found. If she must dig or change the litter, she should wear gloves and wash her hands thoroughly after she's done. If your cat spends time outdoors, she should wash her hands after handling the feline.

GEAR DADDY

If your idea of a good time is shopping for and spending money on items you never knew existed, let alone thought you'd ever find space for in your home, you're going to really dig pregnancy and parenthood. Here's your chance to compare prices on diaper receptacles designed to contain the smell of week-old baby bowel movements, devices that warm baby wipes so they're not bracingly cold when they contact the infant's behind, and other esoteric contraptions.

Some items are absolute necessities. Others you may view as exceedingly superfluous. Say your woman "absolutely needs" a white-noise machine designed specifically to soothe infants to sleep. It may occur to you that her quest for that apparatus is merely a good excuse to go shopping or to keep pace with a pregnant peer who just purchased said item. Your feelings on the matter are largely moot, however. If buying it seems that important to her, don't dispute whether it's a necessity (unless you are on a tight budget, which can actually be a blessing in disguise because it simplifies many purchasing decisions).

Shopping for baby-related items can turn into a full-day odyssey that tests your patience and the limits of your credit card. These marathon mall sessions may also conflict with your weekend sports-viewing routine. But the bottom line is, if your woman wants you to come along, come along you must. Not only can you be helpful carrying heavy items and evaluating the relative merits of two hundred- versus three hundred-thread-count sheets for the cradle, you'll also be demonstrating your desire to be a full partner in pregnancy. You may not have a preference about the kind of nightlight used in the baby's room (those employing an open flame should be avoided for safety's sake), but you will be best off hiding any indifference you may feel.

Here are some of the larger items likely to appear on your prenatal shopping list:

CRADLE AND BEDDING

CRIB AND BEDDING

CHANGING TABLE

DIAPER CONTAINER

STROLLER

BABY JOGGER

BABY BACKPACK and/or **CHEST PACK**

CAR SEAT and related mounting equipment

DIAPER BAG

ROCKING CHAIR

BREAST PUMP (one machine you'll definitely want to see in action)

Many of the above items require assembly and/or installation. Since you are a full partner in this pregnancy venture, those are tasks you also will be expected to perform. Here it is critical that you develop an ability to follow instructions written in fragmentary English by people who obviously have zero grasp of the English language.

WOMB TO ROOM

As a budding middle school student, while making the awkward transition from caveboy to caveman, Gronk discovered during home economics class that he possessed a passion and a flair for interior decorating. While other buddies embraced the rudimentary weapon-production possibilities of woodshop and metalshop, Gronk secretly yearned to immerse himself in color schemes, fabrics, and feng shui. Rather than nurture that passion, however, he buried it in order to avoid ridicule from his peers.

With your woman carrying a baby who eventually will need a properly decorated room of his or her own, here's your chance to finally unfurl your true colors by putting your exquisite interior design eye to good use. You and your woman will most likely end up spending a good deal of time with

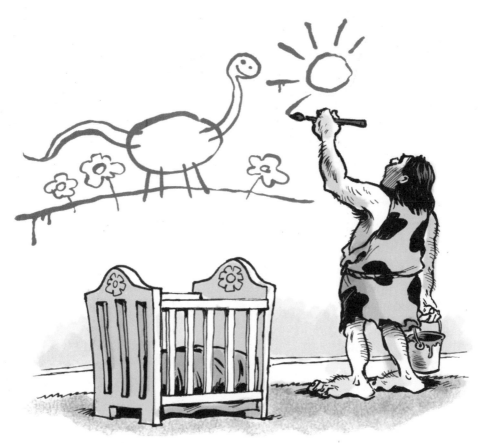

your child in this room, rocking the restless infant to sleep, reading stories, singing lullabies, and changing diapers, so the space needs to be comfortable and engaging without being too crowded or overstimulating. Disco balls, Day-Glo paint, and a surround-sound stereo system probably should wait until the teenage years.

As you work together to create a lively but soothing nursery environment, remember, you will be doing the heavy lifting and equipment assembly. Also, any nursery-related projects involving exposure to fumes from paints, finishes, and the like are yours and yours alone. When it comes to exposure to potentially toxic materials, it's up to you to take one for the team.

Here are a few other key considerations in preparing the baby nursery:

- As you'll come to learn, sleep is of paramount importance and the sleeping habits of parents and child are inextricably linked. So if you have an option of **which room to use as the nursery**, choose one situated in a relatively quiet part of the house. While some infants can sleep through a lot of racket, others are light sleepers who need to be protected from potentially intrusive noises such as the caveman's John Bonham-like basement drumming sessions and buzz-saw snoring.

- Whether you already know the sex of your baby or you're going to wait to find out at delivery, your choice of **color schemes** for the nursery is limitless. Your caveman sensibilities may tend toward earth-tone finishes, perhaps even un-

treated wood, rough-hewn granite, or fieldstone, but these might not be the best options. Instead, let your woman weigh in, then choose from among more practical options—shades of pink, blue, green, purple, and yellow tend to be popular.

- As the parent of an infant who cannot yet crawl or walk, you are sure to pass many hours on the floor, down at rug rat level. Here again, your caveman proclivities shine through; you favor an earthen floor for the nursery. That not being a feasible option, consider a **rug or carpet** that's soft but not so shaggy that the piling envelops the baby.

- Many a parent has discovered the benefits of the **white noise** provided by a small appliance such as a humidifier or dehumidifier. If your infant is easily awakened by noises outside the nursery, try white noise.

- A **changing table** is one of those items you may be able to procure secondhand from a friend or family member whose baby-producing days are over. Whether you get one new or used, it should be sturdy enough to withstand a regular pounding, with a changing surface that's washable (for reasons that will become obvious once you attempt to change the diaper of a kicking, screaming child). The best changing tables are those with plenty of storage space for things you'll readily need: wipes, diapers, ointments, washcloths, towels, etc.

- The same applies with a **crib**. Look for a durable and functional one with all its parts and hardware present and accounted for, keeping in mind your first child may not be the only one who will use it. Also ask people you know whose kids have graduated to beds if they have a crib they'd like to sell. Good, solid cribs and changing tables also can be found at yard sales.

▶ You are a sentimental type, so you want the nursery to have a touch of the cave-like environment to which you were accustomed as a child. But bats, moss, stalactites, and stalagmites aren't suited to an indoor setting. Instead, look to **window coverings** to capture that cave feeling. Shades made of a thick cloth (or other material) that, when drawn, let little light pass through may be just the ticket. However, while darkness does tend to encourage an infant to sleep more soundly, we're not talking sensory deprivation here. No need to go to extremes such as bricking up windows or using blackout shades. You're not raising an infant Eddie Munster; you're raising a child for whom regular glimpses of sunlight are a healthy thing. On the other hand, you don't want your child's sleep affected by tissue-thin window dressings that block no light at all. Find a nice middle ground.

▶ A **rocking chair** is another item that's indispensable and easy to find second-hand. Look for one that is sturdy, roomy enough for man or woman plus baby, cushioned in the seat, and not too creaky.

▶ Decorate the room with **wall adornments and other accoutrements**, but no animal busts, please. There are better spots for your hunting trophies than the baby's

nursery. Stuffed animals are fine, but not the kind you find at the taxidermist. Colorful posters or prints depicting trains, animals (in nonthreatening postures), balloons and the like work well, as do mobiles, nonpoisonous plants, and other items that engage the infant's senses.

▶ Complete the room with **other items**, such as a portable stereo and some good child-oriented music to play on it; a book of lullabies and songs to sing to baby; a nightlight.

PREHISTORIC, YET PROACTIVE AND PROTECTIVE

Your to-do list just keeps getting longer. But that's OK because idle hands are the sign of an idle mind. Here are a few other tasks for the can-do caveman to take care of before the baby arrives:

▶ Test all **smoke alarms** to confirm they are in working order.

▶ Get a **cell phone** so your pregnant woman can reach you at a moment's notice. Make sure it's powered on, fully charged, and you know how to use it, lest you miss the only call that really matters: the one telling you it's time to go to the hospital, OK!

▶ Confirm with your **health insurance** carrier that your child will be covered as part of your plan and adjust your policy as needed. If you don't have health insurance, it's time to join the ranks of responsible adults and get it.

▶ If you don't have insurance, look into enrolling in a **state government** children's insurance program. Every state has insurance programs for infants, children, and teens that are available at little or no cost to parents. You can call (877) Kids Now to learn more.

▶ Establish a **fire-escape route** out of your home, just in case. As you know, cavemen and fire can be a dangerous combination. Confirm that all locks and doors around the house are in good working order and fix any that aren't.

▶ Find a **pediatrician** or family physician for your infant. Your baby likely will be due for a doctor's visit within twenty-four hours of birth (usually while you are still at the facility where he or she was born) and for a host of scheduled and unscheduled visits throughout his or her first year, for checkups, vaccinations, and treatment when ill. Ask friends and family for references, then visit at least a few pediatricians to find one who seems qualified, friendly, and reasonably priced, and who works in a clean, hospitable environment and is supported by a sharp staff. Get a feel for their medical philosophies to determine whether they jibe with yours.

▶ Buy or assemble a home **first aid kit**. Ask your new pediatrician, a family doctor, or other medical professional about which items to include.

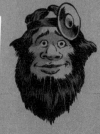

DR. BRIAN

LEARN INFANT CPR ASAP

Quick thinking and decisive action are the hallmarks of a more advanced caveman. Each is absolutely necessary in situations when you may be called on to administer CPR (cardiopulmonary resuscitation) to an infant. This process entails performing rescue breathing to get oxygen to the child's lungs and chest compressions to keep blood circulating.

If an infant's breathing or heartbeat has stopped (due to choking, suffocation, or some other cause), every second counts. These kinds of emergencies are every parent's nightmare, so do your best to avoid them by preparing yourself and your partner to perform CPR. You'll gain peace of mind in knowing you have the skills to revive a child in dire need. It is necessary know-how you hope you never have to put into practice.

Knowing how to do CPR for adults does not mean you know how to perform it on an infant. Because a baby's body is more fragile than an adult's, you need to take extra precautions and use less force in administering infant CPR than you would trying to revive an adult or even an older child.

It's important to point out that simply reading the steps below does not qualify you as an expert on infant CPR. Groups such as the American Heart Association and the American Red Cross recommend that *all* infant caregivers—including parents and babysitters—take a class in CPR for infants. Both organizations offer CPR training classes at the local level. Visit their websites at www.americanheart.org and www.redcross.org to find out about classes in your area.

If an infant isn't breathing, has no apparent pulse, and is not responding:

- Send someone to call 911; however, if you're alone with the child, don't leave him or her alone.

- After performing CPR for one minute according to the steps below, call 911, carrying the infant with you to the nearest phone. If you suspect spinal injury, however, do not move the child.

- Carefully position the child on his or her back. If you suspect a spinal injury, it likely will take two people to move the infant because it is *imperative* you avoid twisting the head or neck.

- Open the child's air passage by lifting the chin with one hand while pressing down on the forehead with the other.

- Is the child breathing? Place your ear near his or her mouth and nose, watch the chest, and feel for breath on your cheek.

- If you do not detect breathing, cover the infant's mouth and nose tightly with your own mouth while ensuring the chin is lifted and the head tilted. (If you suspect a spinal injury, rather than tilting the infant's head back, place your fingers on his or her jaw, touching each side of the head. Now lift the jaw forward gently with your fingers on either side of the head.)

- Slowly breathe two breaths into the infant's air passage, making sure they are neither too large nor too forceful. If you see no rise in the chest, repeat the chin lift, head tilt, and two-breath process (unless you suspect a spinal injury, in which case you will move the jaw as instructed above instead of tilting the head).

- If that doesn't restore breathing, see if something is blocking the airway and try to remove it. A flashlight can help you spot a blockage.

- Still no indication of circulation (normal breathing, coughing, or movement)? Then begin chest compressions. Place two or three fingers on the infant's breastbone, just below the nipples, taking care not to press on the very end of the breastbone. Your other hand should rest on his or her forehead so the head remains tilted back.

- Press down on the infant's chest until it compresses about one-third to one-half the full depth of the chest. Perform a total of five compressions, allowing the chest to rise completely after each and counting each one off. Don't pause between the compressions.

- Now give the infant one slow, full breath as you did earlier. The chest should rise.

- Continue the cycle: five chest compressions, then one breath.

- After a minute, look again for signs of circulation. If you still cannot detect normal breathing, movement, or any other signs of respiration or circulation, now is the time to leave the infant and call 911 for emergency medical assistance.

- After making the call, return to the infant to repeat the compression and breath cycle until the infant recovers or help arrives.

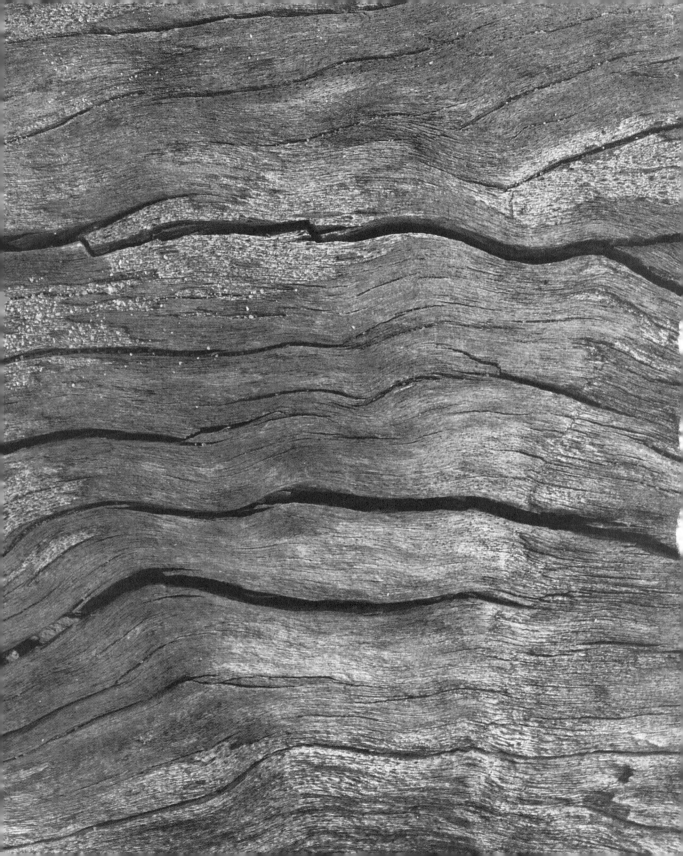

CHAPTER 4

DR. STRANGEGLOVE & THE MEDICAL MYSTERY TOUR

....

The only thing we have to fear is fear itself—nameless, unreasoning, unjustified terror which paralyzes needed efforts to convert retreat into advance.

—FRANKLIN D. ROOSEVELT

....

If men could get pregnant:

A. Natural childbirth would be obsolete.

B. Morning sickness would rate as the nation's number one health problem.

C. All methods of birth control would be improved to 100-percent effectiveness.

D. Children would be kept in the hospital until they were toilet trained.

E. They would not think twins were quite so cute.

F. They would stay in bed for the entire nine months.

G. All of the above.

The correct answer is: *(g) All of the above.* That should come as no surprise to contemporary cavemen, many of whom would just as soon saw off or gnaw off one of their own

GROW WITH GRONK

What the caveman stands to gain from reading Chapter 4:

▶ **THE POWER** to overcome his medical phobias

▶ **ENTRÉE** into the exclusive realm of prenatal caregivers

▶ **A WORKING KNOWLEDGE** of the female reproductive system

▶ **INSIGHT** into how the pregnancy happened in the first place

▶ **AN AWARENESS** of potential birthing venues

▶ **A KNOWLEDGE** of common conditions and maladies that may affect a pregnant woman

▶ **ANSWERS** to fundamental health questions confronting the expectant couple

▶ **INSIGHT** into the medical checkups, tests, and procedures to which a pregnant woman is subjected

▶ **A KNOWLEDGE** of medicines and drugs a woman can safely take during pregnancy

▶ **THE ABILITY** to identify items that are potentially toxic to woman and baby

▶ **A GRASP** of the special health issues associated with pregnant women over age thirty-five

limbs as seek medical attention. Indeed, for cavemen like Gronk, even the remote mention of any form of medical intervention beyond a Band-Aid can conjure the "nameless, unreasoning, unjustified terror" to which F.D.R. referred in his 1933 inaugural speech.

That sense of terror can grip the caveman even when it's his woman and not himself who needs medical attention. A pregnant woman may have as many medical appointments in nine months as a medically phobic caveman will have in a decade or more.

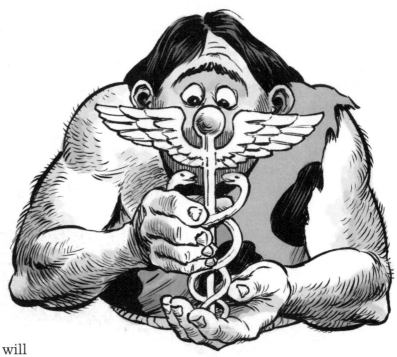

But as an equal partner in the pregnancy venture, it is incumbent on the caveman to overcome his urge to cower from modern medicine and stand tall by assuming an active role in his woman's prenatal care. He can take comfort in knowing that, outside of a few bad apples (Drs. Frankenstein and Moreau, Nurses Ratchet and Diesel, to name several), the medical community is there to help him, not do him harm, when he and his woman are expecting a child.

Most men are somewhat queasy about medical matters. Unlike women, who grow accustomed to seeing doctors for up-close-and-personal routine exams, young, healthy men don't accrue many frequent-patient miles at the doctor's office. When they think about healthcare, many guys only know that at some point in the distant future (is it forty or fifty?) a doctor is going to put his or her finger in a very uncomfortable place, and he or she may even want to stick a camera in there! Many a young man's policy toward medicine could thus be described as "don't ask, don't tell."

Given that mindset, it's not surprising that the whole medical aspect of pregnancy causes fear and anxiety. Pregnancy is particularly petrifying to some men because it is chock-full of fear's two main ingredients: the unknown and a lack of control. Unfortunately, when faced with a fearful situation, the less-evolved members of the male species have a limited range of responses. For them it's either fight or take flight.

And so it is with pregnancy. Some guys fight the process; they are obsessive about the health of woman and baby, perceiving even the most minor symptom as a possible threat. They get so enmeshed in the process that they almost expect they should feel the baby move. Other guys take flight, preferring to let their pregnant partner deal with her "condition" on her own, an out-of-site, out-of-mind attitude that basically amounts to a grown man curling into the fetal position when the going gets tough. These men rationalize their behavior by reasoning that they really can't do much for the pregnant woman anyhow. But a pregnant woman doesn't need or deserve a man who is OCD, ADD, or MIA. She may not say it, but if the only options the caveman brings to the table are fight or flight, his woman will probably start wondering why she agreed to share a cave with him in the first place.

Fortunately, a little knowledge can go a long way toward alleviating the fear of the unknown. And while you can't ever really control the course of a pregnancy, at least you can find out the areas of prenatal health-care where you can be a positive influence, letting the other stuff unfold as it may.

The purpose of this chapter is not to make you a medical expert, but rather to familiarize you with some of the medical basics of pregnancy so that, arm-in-arm with your woman, you can stroll confidently and fully upright into the doctor's office or labor and delivery room.

THE PREGAME SHOW: VIEWER DISCRETION ADVISED

Your daddy said I took you just a little too far
You're telling me things, but your girlfriend lied
You can't catch me 'cause the rabbit done died (yes it did)

—AEROSMITH, "SWEET EMOTION"

We're not going to touch the third rail by weighing in on whether life begins at conception, but it's safe to say that a pregnancy does. So if you and your partner are really going to be responsible about a healthy pregnancy, there are important matters to consider before conception. Chances are, if you are reading this book, you already know there's a baby in your future, so this advice may come a little late. But it does apply to any future pregnancies.

From a medical perspective, the effort to have a healthy pregnancy starts even before a couple realizes they are expecting. The first few weeks of pregnancy, before an early pregnancy test confirms there's a bun in the oven, are crucial to a developing caveling, so a woman who, in anticipation of becoming pregnant, is already getting the right vitamins and nutrition while avoiding drugs and alcohol will be laying the foundation for a healthier, safer pregnancy term.

Consider a typical scenario: woman misses period; woman waits a few days to see if it comes, then when in doesn't, purchases a home pregnancy test kit; the result is positive; woman places a call to caveman who planted said seed; the pregnancy clock is now ticking. In truth, that clock actually started ticking at least two weeks earlier, about two weeks after the woman's last regular period. This is the reason pregnancy and expected delivery dating is based on the LMP, or Last Menstrual Period, as opposed to the CMP, or Cave Man Phone call. At this point the expectant couple will retrace their footsteps to pinpoint their whereabouts when conception occurred. Ah yes, it was that fateful night of wine-fueled Dionysian high jinks on the bearskin rug (see Dr. Brian's Instant Replay below, for a look at how conception unfolds, from a purely clinical perspective, of course).

A woman who is resolved to get pregnant should talk to her doctor about taking **prenatal vitamins** before conception. In

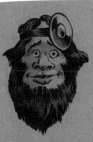

DR. BRIAN

INSTANT REPLAY

Paleolithic sex partners probably had neither the capacity for small talk nor the patience to engage in petting and other forms of what we now call foreplay. Thus, we can surmise that their sexual encounters most closely resembled those we might witness on a television nature program or at the local dog park. While the mating dances leading up to conception are perhaps much different today than they were in prehistoric times, the biological processes associated with conceiving a baby have remained constant. Here's a behind-the-scenes look at the sperm-meets-egg miracle:

- After consuming a candlelit meal of free-range bison and fermented firewater, man escorts woman to comfortable corner of lair.

- Couple cuddles under warm pelts as primal music pulses from the stereo.

- They do the horizontal cave rock, with the man climaxing in an ejaculation of some 300 million sperm, which enter the vagina at a speed of up to 500 centimeters (200 inches) per second.

- By now, the former guardian of those sperm is fast asleep and snoring contentedly. But in a scene with a startling resemblance to the start of the Ironman Triathlon, his little swimmers, propelled forward by flagella, hurtle en masse toward the egg.

- Mucus at the opening of the cervix, normally thick, becomes thinner at the time of a woman's ovulation, allowing some sperm to pass.

- The most intrepid and fortunate of the 300 million swimmers reach the womb, then into the fallopian tubes. At least one egg resides in one of the tubes, leaving sperm at another crossroads.

- A sperm makes a correct tubal turn, contacting an egg, then burrows through the egg's outer wall. When this occurs, the egg's wall becomes impermeable to the other contestants in the race.

- In rare instances, a single egg splits after fertilization, each half developing into an identical fetus, while in other similarly infrequent cases, two eggs are released at the same time and each is fertilized by a separate individual sperm. The former results in identical twins and the latter in nonidentical twins.

- Genetic material from the egg and sperm are joined. What once was just a twinkle in the caveman's eye is now an embryo.

particular, she's going to need an adequate amount of **folic acid**, a B vitamin, to support development of the fetal nervous system early in pregnancy. Prenatal vitamins contain the recommended amount of folic acid, as well as other important vitamins and minerals, such as calcium and iron. Unfortunately, many women don't get started on prenatal vitamins until their first doctor's visit, but by that time they may be a month or more into the pregnancy. It's nothing to stress out about, but bottom line: planning ahead for a pregnancy is best, but if one develops unexpectedly, a woman should promptly start treating her body like the temple (and factory) it is by calling the doctor right away to get a prescription for prenatal vitamins.

MEET THE TEAM

If an errant spear glanced a Cro-Magnon hunter's flesh, he would go to his clan's healer for an herbal poultice remedy and bandage. If a scramble up a steep ledge led to a two-story tumble and a broken limb for a Cro-Magnon gatherer, she would go to the healer—who also happened to be a shaman—for a splint and a spell to chant for quick recovery. When heading off to battle, the Cro-Magnon warrior would visit the same healer/shaman for an amulet to ward off evil spirits; before the warrior left, the shaman would drink a small amount of his blood to give him extra strength.

Evidence left by our prehistoric forebears shows that cave-dwelling caregivers were capable of certain primitive medical pro-

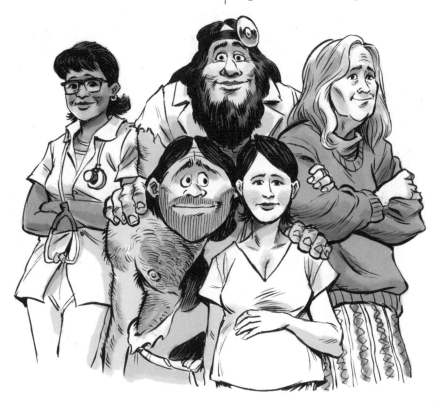

cedures, even brain surgery that involved drilling a hole in the patient's skull to cast out evil spirits (or just relieve a headache). But it was only relatively recently that childbirth became safer. The human head at birth was roughly as big 10,000 years ago as it is today, so childbirth was a risky proposition indeed for mother and baby. Today it is a much safer endeavor, however, thanks to modern medicine, advanced treatment techniques, and skilled care.

The Paleolithic healer did the best he could with the primitive tools at hand. But despite his best efforts, many heroic Cro-Magnon women likely died from childbirth.

Doctors, nurses, midwives, and doulas are to the modern women of today what shamans, healers, and medicine men were to the Cro-Magnon of the Stone Age. If this is your first pregnancy, it's a good bet that you and your partner are going to be meeting a host of these medical professionals over the course of the prenatal period. Since these people are going to play a major role in the coming months in attending to the health of the expectant mother and baby, it's worth finding people with whom you and your partner are comfortable. Too often people make more of an effort choosing someone to work on their car or house than they do choosing someone to work on their body.

Your choice of healthcare providers may be somewhat restricted by your insurance plan. But even if you have a plan with a defined network of providers, you still should have some options within that net-work. When weighing those options, try applying the same principles you use in evaluating other service providers: reputation, convenience, and ideally, someone with whom you feel comfortable. In choosing the professionals to add to your prenatal health team, you may need to solicit advice and referrals from people you trust: recent parents, pregnant moms, and trusted healthcare providers.

In selecting a doctor to provide prenatal care, keep in mind you may also be choosing the group with which that provider works. In that case, the pregnant woman may have a primary doctor she sees regularly, but she also may receive care from other caregivers in the group. Your choice of doctors also will be determined in part by the birthing venue: hospital, home, or birthing center. Certain providers will have "privileges" to work at certain institutions.

Here's a look at some of the key players on the prenatal healthcare team roster:

OBSTETRICIAN-GYNECOLOGIST (OB-GYN).

As doctors who specialize in the care of women, they lead the activities of the medical support team. The obstetrics part of the name refers to pregnancy-related healthcare, while gynecology is the area of medicine dealing with the treatment of women's health, particularly issues related to the reproductive organs. There are also subspecialists within the field of OB-GYN who practice maternal-fetal medicine and these doctors may be consulted in certain high-risk pregnancies.

OB-GYNS are doctors with at least four additional years of training after medical school in women's health and reproduction, including both surgical and medical care. They can handle complicated pregnancies and can also perform cesarean sections. Look for obstetricians who are board-certified, meaning they have passed an examination by the American Board of Obstetrics and Gynecology. Some board-certified obstetricians go on to receive further training in high-risk pregnancies. These physicians are called maternal-fetal specialists, or **perinatologists**.

FAMILY PHYSICIAN. Family-practice doctors train to care for a broad range of health issues in both men and women, young and old. They also train in obstetrics, so they may be your partner's doctor throughout the pregnancy. A family physician who cares for pregnant women will often be the baby's doctor as well, thus the term "family" doctor.

NURSE MIDWIFE. Midwives provide care for women during pregnancy, labor, and delivery. They have different classifications depending on their training. Generally midwives care for low-risk pregnancies, and they will consult with or refer a physician if complications arise. Midwives often work with a physician group, supplementing the prenatal care offered by doctors in the group. According to the U.S. Centers for Disease Control and Prevention (CDC), the percentage of all births attended by midwives has increased steadily since the mid-1970s, from less than 1 percent to about 8 percent. The vast majority (about 95 percent) of midwife-attended births in the United States involve certified nurse midwives (CNMS), registered nurses who have a graduate degree in midwifery, meaning they are trained to handle normal, low-risk pregnancies and deliveries. About three-quarters of midwife-attended births occur in hospitals, according to the CDC. Most CNMS deliver babies in hospitals or birth centers, although some do home births.

THE BIRTHING VENUE

Where will your baby be when he or she takes that magical first breath? Here's another choice the two of you must make. The vast majority of babies—about 99 percent—are born in a hospital, according to the CDC, a rate that has held steady over the past several decades. Among the 1 percent of births that occur outside a hospital, about two-thirds (65 percent) take place in a residence, according to the CDC, while 27 percent occur at a freestanding birthing center. That leaves about 8 percent of nonhospital births unaccounted for. Those presumably are the ones like Gronk's, which occur outdoors or somewhere "afield."

While most births happen in a hospital, you have other options when it comes to birthing venues, each with its own distinct environment and desired outcome.

PONDER THIS

CAN-DOULA

The term **DOULA** (pronounced doo-luh) is derived from a Greek word meaning "servant-woman" or "slave." These days a doula is someone the expectant mom hires to stand by her as part of the labor and delivery team—essentially a person whose chief responsibility is to mother the mother-to-be. A doula is a woman who is specially trained to provide emotional support, encouragement, suggestions, and other forms of assistance prior to, during, and just after labor and childbirth. Ultimately, she is there to help the mother have a positive and safe birth experience, working as her advocate, interacting with other members of the labor and delivery squad, coaching the woman, and attending to her needs. Does the presence of a doula make the caveman's role obsolete? Hardly. In fact, it frees the caveman to be more "in the moment," connecting with and supporting his partner. Having a doula also allows an expectant father to take a breather during the sometimes lengthy labor and delivery process. Those who advocate using a doula even claim having one may shorten first-time labors, decrease the chance of a cesarean section, and lower the need for pain medications and epidural procedures. Most women connect with a doula several months before the baby is due to establish a rapport and a plan for labor and delivery (with the caveman consulting, if he so desires). If you and your partner are considering using one for the upcoming birth, the organization DONA (Doulas of North America) International (www.dona.org) is a good starting point for your search.

HOSPITALS

If your woman is relying on an obstetrician or family practitioner as her primary prenatal care provider, chances are you're planning to have the child in a hospital. As medical facilities, hospitals typically have the equipment and specialized staff to deal with just about any labor and birth issue, expected or unexpected. However, policies, techniques, and environments differ from hospital to hospital, so look for one that serves your needs and desires. These days, hospitals, recognizing couples have varying expectations for their birthing experience, have grown more flexible in what they offer expectant couples. They range from private birthing suites that house you during labor, delivery, and recovery, and that have a rooming-in option, in which the baby stays with mom rather than in the nursery, to water-birthing capabilities and a broader open-door policy for friends and family to attend a birth.

BIRTHING CENTER

Expectant couples who are concerned about the rates of cesarean section, episiotomy, and epidural anesthesia at hospital birthing units may turn to a birthing center, where caregivers stress births that use no induction techniques, no fetal monitoring devices (other than ultrasound), no C-sections or pain-relief drugs (other than a "local" to stitch a perineum tear), and very few episiotomies. Thus, they cater to women who are considered to have low-risk pregnancies and who prefer minimal intervention in the natural childbirth process. While a midwife typically is a key caregiver at a birthing facility, most facilities also have in-house medical support, including nurses and medical equipment. Women who are expecting a multiple birth or a breech birth might not be good candidates for a birthing center; likewise, those who have been diagnosed with preeclampsia or gestational diabetes. In evaluating birth centers, look for one that is accredited by the Commission for the Accreditation of Birth Centers (CABC). The organization's website (www.birthcenters.org) provides a good starting point for your search.

HOME BIRTH

For true homebodies who prefer childbirth to happen in the most familiar of surroundings, there's the home birthing option. The logic goes that a pregnant woman who labors and delivers at home will be more comfortable and relaxed. Home births, like births that occur at birthing centers, are for women with low-risk pregnancies and a desire for minimal intervention. Here again, a midwife tends to be the main care provider, with the expectant couple arranging for standby medical support if the need arises. The Archie Bunker-type caveman may be concerned his woman will choose his favorite recliner as her birthing venue. Don't fret—with the money you're likely to save birthing at home instead of at the hospital, you can buy a brand-new recliner.

ANATOMY 101

Being a proactive partner in pregnancy demands that the caveman become versed in the workings of the female body—and the various components of her reproductive system in particular. A guy who heads into the lengthy procession of medical visits to come without an in-depth knowledge of his woman's relevant parts is flying blind. But the guy who makes an effort to reeducate himself about the relevant components of the female anatomy, which he was first introduced to many years ago in health class, will be an enlightened partner during the journey ahead.

The modern caveman may find it intimidating to talk openly, in clinical terms, about the female reproductive system, especially when the discussion involves people he barely knows or has only recently met. He's not sure how the system works, just that it feels great to be a welcome visitor there. But in accompanying his woman on prenatal medical visits, it behooves him to have some grasp of how the female plumbing functions and the terminology used to describe those functions. While speaking in scientific terms about the holiest of holy places may take some of the mystery out of your intimate conjugal explorations, it will better prepare you for the grand climax of this journey: labor and childbirth.

It also helps if the caveman gets over any irrational anger or resentment he harbors toward his woman's caregivers because

DR. BRIAN

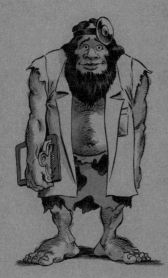

DATE WITH DESTINY

Today you can go to a store and buy a six-pack of beer that specifies the exact date when the beer was conceived at the brewery. It takes a simple mathematical formula for a medical provider to estimate the conception date and project a birth date for a baby. Though only about 5 percent of women deliver on their actual due date, it is nonetheless useful to know how much time you have before the pterodactyl arrives. The doctor typically will trace conception back to the first day of the last menstrual period and make calculations from there. Take that date, add seven days, then count back three months to arrive at a rough due date. That formula for calculating a baby's due date actually overestimates the length of pregnancy, since conception occurs about fourteen days after the first day of the period. But based on this method of calculation, the normal length of a pregnancy is forty weeks. For cavemen who live only in the moment, that's equivalent to 403,200 minutes.

they have full access to body parts he views as his sole domain. Most women are accustomed to having a doctor peer at those parts at least once a year. But for the medically phobic and territorial caveman, the concept of his woman granting unfettered access to her private parts to virtual strangers can be unsettling, especially when his own access may be restricted.

Get over it, guy, because your woman's medical support team will be watching several of her parts very intently during the gestation process. Let's briefly describe them.

The **uterus**, often referred to as the womb, is the strongest muscle in a woman's body. It needs every ounce of strength it can muster to perform the crucial functions of housing the amniotic sac, placenta, and fetus during pregnancy. It's roughly the shape of a light bulb. At the bottom tip of the uterus is the **cervix**. If the uterus is the light bulb, the cervix is its metal screw end. It has a small opening that during labor and delivery thins out (effaces) and opens (dilates). This is one thing doctors (or nurses and midwives) "check" when performing an exam with their fingers inside the vagina.

The **ovaries** and **fallopian tubes** ("tubes" for short) are where eggs are produced and released, usually once a month during ovulation. Typically an ovary releases an egg in the middle of a woman's twenty-eight-day menstrual cycle. For the next few days, the egg is ready to be fertilized. Thus, having intercourse between days twelve to sixteen of the cycle is most likely to cause conception, at which point the egg travels down the fallopian tubes, into the uterus.

The **vagina** is familiar territory for many males, but they know it more as an entry than an exit. This is the opening, made of incredibly strong, resilient tissue, through which the baby passes at birth.

The **placenta** is a round, spongy organ that forms along the walls inside the uterus. It is connected to the fetus by the umbilical cord, through which it provides the baby nourishment. The placenta also acts as a barrier to protect the fetus from toxins.

If you hearken back to your first sex-ed lessons in health class, you'll recall the male gym teacher who taught the class (one of your early caveman mentors) pointing out other prominent parts of the female plumbing. The **perineum**? In females, it's the area directly between the bottom of the vaginal opening and the anus. And what about the **labia minora** and **labia majora**? The outer, larger lips of the vulva are the labia majora, the smaller, more delicate inner lips are the labia minora. **The vulva**? It's the all-encompassing term for the external portion of female genitalia. The **clitoris** is the small, sensitive "button" at the top of the vulva. Your high school gym teacher may not have lingered too long in the description and functions of this important part of the female anatomy. If its "functions" are a mystery to you, consider further research in books devoted specifically to sex. Thus endeth the refresher lesson on the female anatomy.

THE MEDICAL MYSTERY TOUR: PRENATAL CARE

On average, a pregnant woman will make between seven and eleven visits to her prenatal care provider throughout her term. That's about one visit per month. Expectant fathers typically are more than welcome to attend these prenatal visits, although they aren't often present in the room while their woman is being examined.

Your schedule may be such that you cannot join your woman for all the appointments. But by accompanying her to some of them, you're not only taking an active role in the pregnancy partnership, you may also be helping to calm her nerves and provide the kind of support only you can offer. Some of these visits you're not going to want to miss anyway, because they will give you the chance to hear the fetal heartbeat for the first time, to view an image of the baby in the womb via an ultrasound, and to hear from

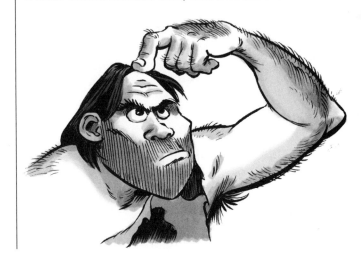

the experts how your little one is developing in its private uterine cave.

Curious what happens during these physical exams? Ready or not, we're going to tell you. A routine prenatal visit includes checking the woman's blood pressure, weight, legs (for swelling), and abdomen (to measure the height of the fundus, the upper section of the uterus).

After about twelve weeks, you may be able to hear the baby's heart ("fetal heart tones") with an **ultrasound** device. Actually hearing the beating heart of the baby for the first time can be an emotionally powerful moment, even for stoic Steve McQueen types.

On the first or second visit, a **pelvic exam** is performed, partly to assess the size of the opening of the woman's pelvis. While not perfect, an estimate of the pelvic dimensions can help predict if the baby might have trouble fitting through the pelvic bones. Toward the end of pregnancy, an internal exam may be performed to check the cervix. By now, after so many exams, this one might remind you of passers-by checking a pay phone for change.

Laboratory and radiology tests are also common during pregnancy. A **Pap smear** (used to detect cancer of the cervix) is performed at one of the initial visits. A pregnant woman also will be screened for various sexually transmitted diseases, including HIV, gonorrhea, chlamydia, syphilis, and hepatitis B. A **blood sample** is tested for immunity to rubella. While your woman was probably vaccinated for rubella as a child, it's in the best interests of fetal health to test

her for the disease anyway. A **urinalysis** also is performed to look for protein, glucose, and bacteria, which even if not causing symptoms, can increase the chance of premature, or preterm, labor.

An ultrasound may be ordered to confirm the dates of the pregnancy and to look for any structural abnormalities in the fetus. Pregnancy dating is critical because the age (in weeks) of the pregnancy is used to measure fetal growth and to establish an estimated date of delivery. The best time to get an ultrasound to check dates is between seven and twelve weeks, while the best time to get one to detect structural abnormalities is between eighteen and twenty weeks. Thus, an ultrasound is usually performed sometime between seven and twenty weeks. Here is when you may be afforded your first glimpse of the budding fetal unibrow.

PRENATAL TESTING PREP-COURSE, OF COURSE

More than anything, expectant parents want proof that their baby is developing normally. The first thing Gronk did when he got a close look at the ultrasound image of his gestating progeny was to confirm the little one had one normal eyebrow and the requisite number of digits.

It's comforting to know that the main purpose of prenatal medical care is to offer proof or at least strong evidence that a fetus is developing as it should, and to ensure the outcome of the pregnancy is as healthy as possible. The battery of medical tests to check on the baby's progress begins in the earliest stages of pregnancy. Exactly which prenatal tests depends on several factors, including genetic risks, health risks, and the preferences of the expectant couple. While today's testing choices may seem confusing, the future looks even more complicated now that we have cracked the human genetic code, opening the door to an ever-expanding array of tests that allow us to learn more and sooner. But let's leave that mind-expanding discussion for another time.

Today a handful of tests may be offered as part of routine prenatal screening. It's well worth knowing about these in advance so you and your partner can make informed decisions about whether to have these tests, and to understand the implications of an abnormal result.

DOWN SYNDROME RISK ASSESSMENT

Down syndrome, or Trisomy 21, is the most common genetic disorder. The risk for a baby is about one in a thousand, but increases with advanced maternal age. For pregnant women who are at least thirty-five years old, the Down syndrome rate goes up to one in 250, and by age forty, the risk is about one in a hundred.

Down syndrome is caused by an extra copy of all or part of chromosome 21. The disorder usually causes characteristic physical features, including a flattened face, widely spaced and slanted eyes, and a smaller head size. Mental retardation is also typical, though there are wide variations in mental ability. Other health problems include poor resistance to infection, hearing loss,

gastrointestinal problems, and heart defects.

An ever-expanding group of tests are offered to assess the risk for Down syndrome, and other less common genetic disorders. Screening begins with "non-invasive" tests (no risk to fetus and mother) in either the first or second trimesters, or both. Abnormal results may be followed by "invasive" tests (some risk for fetus and mother).

First Trimester Screening may be offered between ten and thirteen weeks of gestation. It includes an ultrasound and two blood tests. The ultrasound screening measures nuchal translucency by examining an area of fluid behind the baby's neck. If the result is abnormal, it may indicate a chromosomal problem. The blood tests measure human chorionic gonadotropin (HCG), and pregnancy associated plasma protein-A (PAPP-A). Together, these tests detect about 85 percent of cases of Down syndrome, and even a higher rate for the less common genetic disorder Trisomy 18.

Second Trimester Screening is offered between fifteen and twenty weeks. It may be done as an alternative to the first trimester screen, but may also be done in addition to the first screen, referred to as "sequential testing." It usually involves the measurement of four substances in a maternal blood sample: alpha-fetoprotein (AFP), human chorionic gonadotropin (HCG), estriol, and inhibin A. Second trimester screening can predict 80–85 percent of cases of Down syndrome, and about 80 percent of neural tube defects, such as spina bifida or anencephaly.

Whether a health care provider offers

first trimester screening, second trimester screening, or both, is variable. One advantage to the earlier testing is that if the results are abnormal, further testing can be done to confirm or refute the initial test.

INVASIVE TESTING Chorionic Villous Sampling (cvs) and amniocentesis are two invasive tests used to confirm genetic disorders. These tests are 100 percent accurate because they test actual cell genetics, rather than blood markers. However, they also carry some risk to the baby.

Cvs involves the removal of a small amount of placental tissue via a catheter that is inserted either through the abdomen or vagina. In cases where earlier detection of fetal abnormalities is desired, cvs can be performed between nine and fourteen weeks, when the lower volume of amniotic fluid makes amniocentesis more risky. Even so, cvs has a generally higher risk of miscarriage: about one in a hundred.

Amniocentesis is a procedure in which a needle is inserted through a pregnant woman's abdomen, into the space around the fetus, to withdraw a sample of amniotic fluid. The sample then can be analyzed to detect chromosomal abnormalities, neural tube defects, and other genetic diseases, such as cystic fibrosis and sickle cell anemia. The procedure carries a risk of miscarriage of about one in two hundred. Besides identifying potential fetal health issues, the genetic analysis from an "amnio" also can be used to definitively identify the gender of the baby, in case you're interested in knowing ahead of time.

Cvs may be performed as early as ten to twelve weeks gestation, while amniocentesis is generally done between fifteen and nineteen weeks. The earlier detection of problems with cvs allows more time to make the difficult decision of whether to proceed with a pregnancy, but it's complication rate is higher than with amniocentesis. Your health care provider should be able to help you and your partner negotiate these and other complicated pregnancy testing decisions.

OTHER GENETIC DISORDERS There are several other genetic diseases for which screening is offered. Several of these are based on particular high risk populations.

▶ **ASHKENAZI JEWS** The majority of Jewish people in the United States are descended from the Jewish communities of Germany, Poland, Austria, and Eastern Europe. There are a number of diseases that are more common in this population, including Tay-Sachs disease, Canavan disease, familial dysautonomia, and cystic fibrosis. The American College of Obstetricians and Gynecologists (ACOG) recommends screening for, at a minimum, Tay-Sachs disease, Canavan disease, and cystic fibrosis in patients of European-Jewish ancestry.

▶ **AFRICAN-AMERICANS** Sickle cell disease is an inherited disorder that occurs primarily in African-Americans and causes the development of abnormal red blood cells. This leads to anemia (a lack of red blood cells, which carry oxygen to all the body cells) and damage to important body organs. Sickle cell disease is sometimes fatal.

Cystic fibrosis is a genetic condition that causes the body to produce excessively thick, sticky mucus that clogs the lungs and pancreas, impairing breathing and digestion. The disease is carried on a recessive gene, meaning that a person born with one copy of the gene doesn't have the disease. But if two parents are carriers, their child can get both copies, and thus have the disease. Screening is routinely offered to check for the possibility of inheritance of this condition.

CREATURE DISCOMFORTS

Carrying a child in the womb for nine months or so is nothing short of heroic, especially given the many potential health issues that pregnant women must deal with over the course of three trimesters. All the prehistoric procreator can do is stand by and offer support as his woman confronts cardiovascular, gastrointestinal, and neurological/psychological issues, ranging from a queasy stomach to a lack of balance. See p. 74 for a look at some of the most common symptoms and conditions that the sometimes vindictive Hera, Greek goddess of fertility, has been known to inflict upon females, plus some suggestions for finding relief.

FAQ FOR THE FSC
(FREQUENTLY STUMPED CAVEMAN)

There's so much for expectant parents to learn about prenatal health issues and so little time to do so. Here are some of the burning health questions likely to run through a contemporary Cro-Magnon's head when his woman is with child. Keep in mind that some of these head-scratchers involve extremely sensitive subjects and intensely personal decisions that only a discussion between the two of you will resolve. Here's where a caveman's communication skills will really be tested.

SHOULD WE FIND OUT THE SEX OF THE BABY AHEAD OF TIME? There are some benefits to finding out the sex of the baby in the womb. For one, you can focus on girls' names or boys' names and start calling the baby "she" or "he" instead of "it." You may also prepare a bit differently by buying more gender-specific clothing and adjusting the nursery color scheme. Couples who choose to find out the sex of their baby during pregnancy usually get the news from an ultrasound test, which provides detailed images of the baby *in utero*.

But there's something to be said for the old-school route—learning if your baby will be Tong or Tonga in the delivery room, right at birth. There are so few surprises in life, particularly in today's world with instant access to every bit of information. Some people shy from surprises and prefer to get whatever information they can in advance. But sometimes the surprise factor makes the wait even more rewarding, adding excitement, conversation fodder, and mystery to the entire pregnancy.

CAN WE SAFELY HAVE INTERCOURSE WHEN MY WOMAN IS PREGNANT? The term "safe sex" takes on a new meaning during pregnancy. Unless your woman's doctor

WALK A MILE IN HER SHOES: WHY PREGNANCY CAN BE A PAIN

CONDITION/SYMPTOM	RELIEF
NAUSEA/VOMITING	Eating and drinking foods with ginger as an ingredient, such as ginger snaps or ginger ale, may provide relief from nausea. So may eating more frequent but smaller meals. Some women find relief by eating a small snack such as crackers first thing in the morning.
HEMORRHOIDS	Soaking in a bath with Epsom salts can take some of the sting out of those cruel bumps, as can applying witch hazel compresses. Something as simple as avoiding sitting for long periods also helps.
CONSTIPATION	Incorporating whole grains, bran, fresh fruits, and vegetables into the diet can relieve the digestive logjam. So can drinking plenty of fluids, including prune juice, a natural laxative. Exercise may also get her system moving again.
FREQUENT URINATION	Frequent trips to the toilet are the only remedy for this.
LOSS OF LUNG POWER/ SHORTNESS OF BREATH	Sleeping with upper body propped up can allow her to breath easier. Suggest she decrease activity as well.
SCIATIC NERVE PAIN	Stretching and shifting positions can help. So can elevating legs and feet.
BACKACHE	Practicing good posture can help alleviate back pain, as can wearing comfortable shoes (with low or no heel). Some women find relief sleeping on their side rather than back. The caveman can help, too, by providing massage and/or a heating pad.
LACK OF BALANCE	Shifting physical dimensions can give the pregnant woman a new center of gravity and thus, difficulty maintaining balance. Practicing prenatal yoga can help her reclaim lost equilibrium.
FATIGUE/EXHAUSTION	Carrying and providing nourishment to a baby can drain a woman of energy. Rest helps restore it. Exercise and eating healthy also can provide women with an energy boost.
INSOMNIA	Forms of relief may include bathing before bedtime, exercising, practicing deep breathing, and other relaxation methods.
HEARTBURN	Antacids (if cleared for use by doctor) can take away the burn. So can eating smaller, more frequent meals and avoiding spicy, acidic foods and beverages. Lying down immediately after a meal should be avoided.
MUSCLE ACHES/CRAMPS	Massage and stretching can take away the pain.
SWELLING OF EXTREMITIES	Drinking more fluids and spending time in water help curb that bloated feeling.
VARICOSE VEINS	Spending time with legs elevated can alleviate the condition, as can avoiding sitting cross-legged. Some women find wearing support hose helps as well.
HEADACHES	Changing diet, such as increasing iron intake, can relieve headaches. She may also want to try exercising. Over-the-counter pain relievers may work wonders if the doctor clears her to take them.

determines having intercourse puts woman and/or baby at risk—for such conditions as placenta previa, a previous preterm birth, etc.—the only obstacles to sexual activity will be circumstances: lack of energy, lack of interest, preoccupation with pressing baby-related matters, those kinds of things. See the Cava Sutra section of Chapter 5 for hints on maintaining some semblance of a sex life during pregnancy.

CAN A PREGNANT WOMAN RIDE ON AN AIRPLANE? You want to take your woman on a trip before the baby comes and you're wondering whether it's OK for her to fly to your destination. Air travel is fine for her, at least in the first two trimesters, as long as her doctor has found no condition to prevent her from doing so (such as a high risk of preterm labor). Late in the third trimester, her doctor may suggest that she stay close to home and avoid air travel so she can be within close range of her care providers should a condition arise that requires immediate attention. In addition, many airlines restrict women from flying when pregnancy reaches thirty-six weeks (thirty-five weeks for international flights).

CAN MY WOMAN AND I TAKE A HOT TUB TOGETHER? No hot tubbing when she's pregnant, fella. A woman who elevates her body temperature by soaking in a hot tub (or sitting in a sauna) for a sustained period during pregnancy could put the baby at risk. Doctors recommend that an expectant mom's body temperature not exceed 102.2

degrees Fahrenheit for a sustained period of ten minutes or more. A warm bath is fine, but the caveman might not be invited to partake.

IS IT SAFE FOR A PREGNANT WOMAN TO DRINK COFFEE OR OTHER CAFFEINATED BEVERAGES? There's no solid medical data to indicate with any certainty that consuming caffeine in moderation puts the baby at risk. So if she wants a cup of coffee or tea, or a can of cola, there's no clear health reason to deter her from doing so. However, our dietary advisor, Kelli, recommends limiting caffeine intake to about one twelve-ounce coffee (or its equivalent) per day. Also, while herbal teas can be a good substitute and offer warm comfort, avoid those that contain the following: lobelia, sassafras, coltsfoot, comfrey, and pennyroyal. Each of these ingredients carries some possible degree of risk to the mother and baby and should be avoided in any form.

CAN A WOMAN DRINK ALCOHOL DURING PREGNANCY? There are various attitudes about the issue of alcohol consumption by pregnant women. Just a generation previous in the United States, it wasn't unusual for women to drink alcohol during pregnancy without reservation. But today we know that alcohol consumption by an expectant mother certainly provides no fetal benefits; evidence now also strongly suggests that even moderate alcohol consumption puts the health and development of the baby at some type of risk. Because medical science has not determined if there is any safe level of alcohol consumption for pregnant women, many doctors urge—and many women prefer—complete abstinence from alcohol when they are expecting. Some doctors say it's OK for a pregnant woman to occasionally have a drink, particularly if it helps reduce her stress and tension, both of which can be detrimental to the baby. Ultimately, it's a personal decision your woman will make in consultation with you and her health providers.

We'll take a similarly noncommittal stance on alcohol consumption by the expectant caveman, although we can guarantee there will be times during the next nine months when you will want something stronger to drink than water and warm milk.

WHAT POTENTIAL RISKS IS THE BABY EXPOSED TO IF THE MOTHER SMOKES DURING PREGNANCY? Smoking is bad for a person's health, pregnant or not. But when an expectant mother continues smoking during pregnancy, she's endangering the health of the baby. A woman who smokes during pregnancy is less able to provide oxygen to the fetus. A pregnant woman who smokes also is more apt to have a baby with low birth weight, a risky proposition for a newborn. If your woman hasn't quit smoking already, do whatever it takes to get her to stop immediately.

HOW MUCH WEIGHT IS MY WOMAN GOING TO GAIN DURING PREGNANCY? It's healthy, and indeed necessary, for a woman to gain weight during pregnancy. How much she should gain depends on her weight prior to pregnancy. If she's of normal weight, an increase of twenty-five to thirty-five pounds is considered normal and healthy, according to the American College of Obstetricians and Gynecologists. The suggested range is lower for women who were overweight prior to pregnancy and higher for women who were underweight.

SHOULD WE GO FOR A DRUG-FREE "NATURAL" CHILDBIRTH? You are wise to lean heavily on your woman, the one who must endure the pain associated with childbirth, for an answer to this question. Your job is to support whatever decision she makes in consultation with members of the baby-catching team. Some women are resolved to not use pain-blocking or painkilling drugs during labor and delivery. If your woman feels that way, more power to her. Be advised that her resolve may melt away once labor begins.

IF TESTING DETERMINES THERE IS A FETAL DEFECT, HOW DO WE PROCEED? In the rare instance that medical tests reveal some sort of fetal defect, the couple face a heart-wrenching and highly personal decision: to keep or abort the fetus. Our only recommendation is to discuss the possibilities and outcomes among yourselves and with people you trust before making a decision.

IS IT SAFE FOR A WOMAN TO EXERCISE THROUGHOUT PREGNANCY? Regular exercise is good for pregnant women. But she should avoid activity that is so strenuous it elevates her heart rate above levels deemed safe by her medical caregivers (140 beats per minute is the maximum typically recommended during pregnancy) or so dangerous it puts her and the baby at risk. Check out Chapter 5 for suggestions on how the expectant couple can stay (or get) fit during pregnancy.

SHOULD MY WOMAN BREAST-FEED AFTER CHILDBIRTH? Breasts aren't just playthings; they serve a genuine nonsexual function as the main source of nutrition for babies. Our early ancestors breast-fed their offspring for as long as the first two to three years of life or longer. But with the advent of baby formula and new, more modest social customs, breast-feeding became unfashionable in the United States in the mid-twentieth century. Now, however, with medical study after medical study pronouncing its benefits, breast-feeding is back in fashion.

Besides obvious voyeuristic advantages for the caveman, breast-feeding offers tangible benefits to both mother and baby:

- Breast milk provides sugars, fats, and protein that are just right for your baby.
- Breast milk helps keep your baby from getting sick by providing antibodies from the mom to help fight common respiratory and intestinal illnesses.
- Sucking on the breast is good for your baby's jaw and helps future teeth grow straight.
- Growth charts from the World Health Organization indicate that bottle-fed babies have a higher risk of obesity as adults.
- Breast-feeding helps your woman recover from childbirth, encouraging the release of healing hormones.

- Producing milk is a metabolic activity that uses two hundred to five hundred calories a day. So breast-feeding may help her get back her old body faster.
- Mothers who don't breast-feed have been shown in numerous studies to have a higher risk of reproductive cancers.

That said, not all women are able to or wish to breast-feed. Ultimately, it will be up to your woman to decide what's best for her and the baby.

SHOULD OUR BOY BE CIRCUMCISED? A caveman's feelings of sympathetic pregnancy toward his woman quickly transfer to his newborn son when the conversation turns to circumcision. Circumcision is the surgical removal of the fold of skin (foreskin) covering the infant's penis. Determining factors in the decision whether to circumcise tend to be social and cultural. In the United States about 60 percent of boys are circumcised and it is downtrending. It's very common in Islamic as well as Jewish cultures.

The procedure has its purported benefits, namely decreased risk of urinary tract infection and easier hygiene. But since it is a surgical procedure, it comes with risks, too—possible infection and excessive bleeding. This procedure may be painful to the young patient and a local anesthetic may be used. For male witnesses, especially the new dad, it may be excruciating to watch.

Discuss the procedure and all the possible pros and cons with your doctor and ask questions. Then decide for yourselves what you feel is best.

WHAT DO WE DO WITH THE PLACENTA?
Cultures throughout the ages have honored the life-giving force they see embodied in the placenta in their own ways. Some, it is said, even consumed it in a ceremonial context. Even today, there are apparently people who carry on that tradition; a quick Internet search for "placenta recipes" yields hundreds of tasty ways to enjoy the "other red meat." While we applaud the barbarity and pagan possibilities of eating placenta, we will refrain from providing any such recipes in Chapter 6.

HOW IS HER BODY GOING TO CHANGE AFTER CHILDBIRTH? It's common for both members of the expectant couple to experience physical changes from pregnancy. Addressing those changes can be easier for some men than for women. Guys can eliminate the spare tire they've been cultivating during her pregnancy with some regular exercise. For women, however, the aftereffects of her childbearing and delivery room heroics may persist a bit longer.

Many women are left with **stretch marks** around the ribcage, breasts, lower abdomen, hips, and thighs. Here's where the caveman can help by sending her to the day spa, where between the massage, facial, and pedicure, she can consult directly with a skin expert about specific creams, oils, and techniques that may help reduce or eliminate stretch marks. An exercise routine that includes regular abdominal work also can help.

Caused by circulatory issues exacerbated by pregnancy, **varicose veins** are another possible side effect of childbearing. If your woman discovers parts of her legs look like roadmaps, her doctor may send her to a dermatologist. Keeping her legs elevated, wearing support hose, and exercising regularly can alleviate the condition during and after pregnancy.

Then there are the recovery issues that aren't outwardly obvious. As you have found during your field research over the years, the vagina is a strong, resilient, and snugly fitting muscle. Stretched to its limits by a vaginal delivery, it will need extra time to regain its former state. Typically, it will be about six weeks after birth before a woman is cleared by her doctor to have intercourse. Some women snap back into shape quickly and are ready to get back to it depending on whether she had a tear or an episiotomy during delivery. Others need more time and extra rehab. Here's where the caveman can help out by leading his woman through regular Kegel exercises (see p. 112). Doing regular Kegels during pregnancy can help her recover more quickly and make the delivery easier, too. Doing them after childbirth—Kegels typically are the first exercise a woman is cleared to do after delivery—can help her regain that friendly, vise-like grip.

TOXIC BLOCK

Pregnancy can bring out a caveman's most primal protective instincts. Even the most mild-mannered of men has been known to beat his chest, wave his cudgel, and brandish his spear at the faintest sign something is endangering his pregnant woman and baby.

But what happens when the threat is impervious to spear, club, or display of manhood? In this case it's up to the expectant dad to take a more tactful approach by educating himself and his woman about environment toxins—substances, organisms, and physical agents that can produce permanent abnormalities in an embryo or baby. These toxins are called teratogens, and when a pregnant woman is exposed to them, so, too, may be the baby.

The sixteenth-century Swiss physician and alchemist Paracelsus, another in a long line of cultivated cavemen who helped shape history, laid down the guiding principle of toxicology when he said, "The dose makes the poison." But besides dosage, evidence also suggests that timing determines the impact of toxin exposure. During the early stage of fetal organ formation (day eighteen through day sixty of gestation), for example, such exposure can lead to anatomical malformations. Exposure in the second or third trimester may lead to low birth weight, stillbirth, or impaired cognitive development.

As expectant parents, your job is to protect your little one as best you can by avoiding exposure to teratogens.

Here are a few garden variety toxins you're most likely to come across:

ALCOHOL. Women who consume alcohol at a rate of more than two drinks a day have a greater risk of spontaneous abortion. High alcohol consumption also can result in a baby being born with fetal alcohol syndrome, which may involve low birth weight, abnormalities in formation of the cranium and facial structure, and neurological issues, such as decreased IQ. Low-level alcohol consumption does not appear to be a significant risk factor for spontaneous fetal loss. However, because no clear threshold has been established, no amount of alcohol in pregnancy is considered to be safe.

SMOKING. Dr. Brian explains in Chapter 3 about the dangers of secondhand smoke. The effects of firsthand smoke are, of course, even worse for the expectant mom and baby. Smoking during pregnancy not only increases the rate of spontaneous abortion, it can also lead to placenta previa, bleeding during pregnancy, and premature rupture of placental membranes. Smoking is related to low birth weight, a potential difficulty for infants. Exposure to secondhand smoke is directly linked to infant mortality from SIDS.

ORGANIC SOLVENTS. This encompasses a broad range of chemicals (including erchloroethylene, toluene, isopropyl alcohol, acetone, xylene, styrene, and many more) to which an expectant mother and fetus may be exposed through inhalation, skin contact, or ingestion. These potentially harmful solvents can be found in the vapors of items as common as certain kinds of paint, nail polish, gasoline, lighter fluid, and aerosol sprays. In most cases the risk to fetal health increases with exposure to these substances. For example, occasional use of nail polish seems unlikely to constitute a great risk to the baby, as long as exposure time is limited and ventilation is adequate. Chronic exposure may be more harmful, so if your woman is a manicurist by trade, she may want to consider finding a new line of work, at least while she's with child.

LEAD. Exposure to high levels of lead is known to cause embryotoxicity, growth and mental retardation, increased perinatal mortality, and developmental disability. Lead exposure can come from a variety of sources, including lead solders, pipes, storage batteries, lead-based paints, dyes, and wood preservatives. Lead is also one of the most common groundwater contaminants from hazardous waste sites.

SOME OTHER RECOGNIZED HUMAN TERATOGENS. Cocaine, opiates including heroin/methadone, lithium, mercury, radiation from cancer therapy, maternal obesity (severe), vitamin A deficiency, herpes simplex, HIV, syphilis, toxoplasmosis, hyperthermia, and hypoxia.

Knowing as much as you now do about toxins, you must fight the instinct to take radical protective steps such as hermetically sealing your home and quarantining your mate for the duration of her pregnancy. Instead, take a step back and remind yourself that obsessing will get you nowhere.

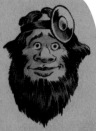

DR. BRIAN

SAFE STUFF

With so many worries about the expectant mother and fetus, the caveman may want to urge his woman to stay indoors and remain immobile for the entire nine-month gestational period. Here are a few items and activities the prehistoric paranoiac and his woman shouldn't have to worry about:

- ▶ **MICROWAVE OVENS**
- ▶ **EXPOSURE TO ELECTROMAGNETIC FIELDS**
- ▶ **CELLULAR TELEPHONES**
- ▶ **DIAGNOSTIC X-RAYS**
- ▶ **HAIR DYE**
- ▶ **USING A HEATING PAD**
- ▶ **SWIMMING IN A POOL**
- ▶ **AIRPORT SCREENING DEVICE**
- ▶ **LIDOCAINE AT THE DENTIST'S OFFICE**
- ▶ **AIR TRAVEL BEFORE THIRTY-SIX WEEKS**
- ▶ **NAIL POLISH REMOVER (IN WELL-VENTILATED SPACE)**
- ▶ **ACCUPUNCTURE TREATMENTS**

Exercise what control you do have over your woman's environment and health, but do so within reason. Cavemen who are especially concerned about warding off toxins can consult their family shaman for suggestions about potential rituals and charms that afford protection to their woman and unborn child.

DISORDERLY CONDUCT: COMMON HEALTH PROBLEMS IN PREGNANCY

As if the expectant caveman weren't feeling paranoid and defensive enough after digesting the previous section about environmental toxins, now he must ponder the possibilities—however slim—of other pregnancy-related health disorders. Now's a good time to reach for a stress-relieving beverage and remind yourself that the majority of expectant couples will have a normal, healthy pregnancy, free of the conditions described below.

Preeclampsia, a.k.a. pregnancy-induced hypertension, is when pregnancy causes a woman to have high blood pressure. In some cases, preeclampsia is preceded by a diagnosis of gestational hypertension, another form of high blood pressure during pregnancy. Hypertensive disorders occur in 12 to 22 percent and preeclampsia in about 5 to 8 percent of pregnancies in the United States. For reasons that have yet to be explained medically, women in their first pregnancies are at higher risk of having such conditions. Women with a family history of high blood pressure during pregnancy face a higher risk of having the condition themselves, as

do women with diabetes, women thirty-five years of age or older, and women who have a prolonged interval between pregnancies. Preeclampsia usually emerges in the second or third trimester. Indications and symptoms include sudden, rapid weight gain and facial edema (swelling), the presence of protein in the urine, low platelets in the blood, anemia, headaches, and blurred vision. If left untreated, it can curb fetal growth and cause a rupture and hemorrhage of the placenta. Treatment usually involves blood pressure medications, bed rest, and/or monitoring both mother and baby closely.

Infections also can be an issue for some women during pregnancy. Among the most common is the **urinary tract infection** (UTI), which is caused by bacteria in the bladder.

An infection may manifest itself as something called **asymptomatic bacteriuria**, in which there is bacterial growth but no symptoms. This is one of the main reasons your woman will undergo routine urine testing at prenatal visits. Left untreated, a UTI and bacteriuria can lead to premature labor. They are typically treated with an oral antibiotic that is safe for the baby. To prevent them, women should drink lots of water, urinate often, especially after sex, and after urinating, wipe from front to back.

Group B streptococci (GBS) is a bacteria that lives in the vaginal or rectal areas of 30 to 40 percent of healthy pregnant women. A woman who has group B strep on her skin is said to be "colonized" with the germ. For every hundred colonized women who have a baby, one or two will have babies infected with the bacteria. Being colonized usually doesn't make the woman sick. It's generally an infected baby that needs treatment. If there is a suspicion the baby is infected, blood cultures will be done and antibiotics may be administered until the diagnosis is confirmed. Doctors usually test for GBS with a swab to the vagina and rectum in the last month of pregnancy. Women who test positive may be prescribed antibiotics at that time, and they usually will be prescribed antibiotics during labor in an attempt to decrease the rate of transmission to the fetus.

Some women are diagnosed with **gestational diabetes** during pregnancy. Diabetes is a condition in which the body has trouble producing or utilizing the hormone insulin, which performs the critical job of converting glucose into energy. During pregnancy, hormones from the placenta can trigger the gestational form of diabetes; women who are over thirty, obese, and/or have diabetes in the family have the highest risk of contracting it. A glucose screening, typically administered by the doctor sometime in the latter part of the second trimester or the early part of the third, is most often used to identify the condition. Mild cases can be treated with diet adjustments and exercise, while more severe cases may require the woman to begin closely monitoring glucose levels and taking insulin. If treated during pregnancy, oftentimes the condition disappears once the baby is born. But a failure to control diabetes during pregnancy can lead to various fetal health issues, including an abnormally large baby or a baby with jaundice, breathing problems, and/or shortages of vital nutrients.

Preterm labor means labor occurring prior to the thirty-seventh week of pregnancy, before the baby is considered fully developed. It occurs in 8 to 12 percent of all births in the United States. Women who are expecting a multiple birth (twins or more), who have had a prior preterm delivery, who smoke or who are either younger than eighteen or older than forty are among those who face a higher risk of preterm delivery. Uterine issues, infections, problems with the placenta, and fetal issues also can cause it. A doctor may address them by prescribing a "tocolytic" medicine to decrease uterine contractions and steroids to hasten development of the baby's lungs, so there is less chance of breathing problems after birth. Bed rest may also be mandated.

Manifested by vaginal bleeding and abdominal or back pain, abruptio placentae, or **placental abruption**, is a separation of the placenta from the site of uterine implantation before birth. The incidence is about one in 150 deliveries. The severe form, which results in fetal death, occurs only in about one out of 500 to 750 deliveries. Causes range from high blood pressure and diabetes during pregnancy to alcohol and drug abuse.

The placenta is an organ that develops in the uterus during pregnancy to nourish the baby. Oxygen and nutrients pass through the placenta to the baby, and waste products pass back out. The condition known as **placenta previa** occurs when the placenta becomes implanted near or over the cervix, thus covering the entry into the vagina from the uterus. The incidence of placenta previa is approximately one in 200 births. When it occurs—usually late in pregnancy—it may cause abnormal, sometimes heavy bleeding, premature separation of the placenta from the uterus, premature birth, and emergency cesarean section. The caveman may not be especially thrilled about the suggested treatments for placenta previa, particularly a prohibition against sexual intercourse. But that may be necessary, as might bed rest, if the condition is serious enough. If bleeding is especially heavy or the pregnancy is at thirty-seven weeks or more, the baby may be delivered, usually by cesarean section.

As many as 20 percent of all pregnancies end before the twentieth week in **miscarriage**. Symptoms may include bleeding and pelvic pain, but not all bleeding means that there will be a miscarriage. Up to 40 percent of women with healthy pregnancies have bleeding in the first trimester due to implantation of the egg in the uterus. The vast majority of miscarriage occurs before the twelfth week, and in general, most pregnancies that reach this point have a good chance of completion. Most miscarriage is caused by a genetic mistake and the fetus doesn't develop properly.

Whatever the causes, a miscarriage may be one of the most difficult times you go through with your partner. It's important for couples to have a discussion with their doctor about the symptoms of miscarriage, and what to do if these symptoms occur.

DR. BRIAN

AT YOUR CERVIX, DEAR: BED REST DURING PREGNANCY

When, in a doctor's judgment, being upright and active threatens the pregnancy and/or the health of a baby, he will urge bed rest, recommending that the woman remain horizontal and relatively inactive until her condition stabilizes or she gives birth. Fortunately, few women have this immobility forced upon them; among those who do, it usually is due to one of the following doctor's diagnoses:

▶ **AN INCOMPETENT CERVIX,** in which the cervix opens too early in term, enhancing the chance of premature birth. Sometimes this is treated with surgery to close the cervix until it is medically safe for the woman to give birth.

▶ **HIGH BLOOD PRESSURE**

▶ **THREATENED MISCARRIAGE,** if the pregnancy is in question or if there is bleeding

▶ **PRETERM LABOR,** when the pregnancy is threatening to end early

Bed rest comes in several forms: modified is basically whatever sort of rest schedule the medical practitioner advises, some being more flexible than others; strict is rigid—usually it means being on the bed or couch and only getting up to use the bathroom; hospital/complete is the strictest and may include hospitalization and prohibition from getting out of bed for long stretches of the day. It may also involve special positioning to alleviate pressure on the cervix.

EXPECTANT MOTHER'S LITTLE HELPERS: MEDICATIONS DURING PREGNANCY

Things are different today,
I hear every mother say
Cooking fresh food for a husband's
   just a drag
So she buys an instant cake, and she burns
   her frozen steak
And goes running for the shelter of a
   mother's little helper
And two help her on her way, get her
   through her busy day
Doctor, please, some more of these
Outside the door, she took four more
What a drag it is getting old

—THE ROLLING STONES,
"MOTHER'S LITTLE HELPER"

Pain and suffering are essential parts of the Human Condition. Much to the chagrin of reproductive-minded women everywhere, pain and suffering also are part of the pregnant condition. Throughout the centuries, shamans, medicine men, healers, alchemists, multinational corporations, and practitioners of modern medicine have quested for ways to quell mankind's pain and suffering.

The result of their quest is what modern man calls drugs and medicines. Today these substances are classified in several broad categories: there are over-the-counter drugs and prescription drugs; some drugs are legal to produce, buy, and consume, others are not. Some medicines come from natural, herbal sources; others are made from synthesized ingredients.

There's also a key distinction to be made between the drugs and medicines that are considered safe for a pregnant woman to ingest—those presenting little or no risk—and those that she should avoid because medical research suggests they pose a considerable risk to her and/or the baby inside her.

Today we have access to a huge array of medicines and remedies that claim to address virtually any imaginable condition. Some of these substances are deemed safe for a pregnant woman to consume; others she should avoid because of the risks they may pose. For a caveman who's never been afraid to try any drug thrust his way, prescription or over-the-counter, legal or otherwise, it may come as a surprise to learn which are considered safe for expectant moms and which are not. So before your woman reaches in the medicine cabinet for meds she had taken often prior to pregnancy, she should now consult her doctor. After reading this section, you'll be able to provide some input as well. That doesn't automatically qualify you as an expert, so be sure she gets some bona fide professional advice.

PRESCRIPTION DRUGS. The U.S. Food and Drug Administration divides prescription drugs into five categories for the purposes of assessing their safety during pregnancy.

CATEGORY A: No demonstrable risk to the fetus in the first trimester; no evidence of risk in later trimesters; possibility of fetal harm appears remote.

CATEGORY B: No confirmed risk in women in the first trimester; no evidence of risk in later trimesters, but animal reproduction studies may have shown an adverse effect.

OVER-THE-COUNTER MEDICATIONS Q & A

QUESTION	ANSWER	NOTES
What's OK for pain, headache or fever?	Acetaminophen (Tylenol) at recommended doses is safe. Aspirin, ibuprofen (Motrin, Advil), and naproxen (Aleve) are not safe unless prescribed by a doctor.	Adult-level doses of aspirin during early pregnancy are linked to possible miscarriage and other complications. Steer clear.
What's safe for allergy symptoms?	Loratadine (Claritin) is considered safe. Diphenhydramine (Benadryl) is safe after the first trimester. Chlorpheniramine maleate or doxylamine are safe throughout pregnancy.	Caution to cavemen: wear protective gear before trying to pronounce these ingredients, and never operate heavy machinery while reading the small type on an item from the pharmacy.
How about congestion and runny nose?	Pseudoephedrine (Pseudofed) is generally safe after the first trimester, but ask the doctor in case there have been any health problems during the pregnancy. Decongestant nasal sprays (Afrin, Dristan) are probably safe, since they are minimally absorbed into the body.	Cold and flu products usually have various combinations of ingredients, so it's best to check the ingredients on the box. Confused about it? Ask the doc.
What can she do about a cough?	Dextromethorphan (the "DM" in Robitussin DM) is safe as directed; guaifenesin is an expectorant (also in Robitussin), and is safe.	Hot non-caffeinated teas with honey can help, but if the cough persists, see the doc.
What about heartburn?	Calcium carbonate (Tums) is safe. Adding magnesium or aluminum hydroxide (Mylanta or Maalox) is OK, too. "H2 blockers" ranitidine (Zantac), cimetidine (Tagamet) and famotidine (Axid) are also considered safe.	It's best not to use antacids at high doses or for prolonged periods. Nizatidine (Axid), another type of H2 blocker, can potentially cause danger to the fetus, so it's not a good choice.
What about intestinal gas? She's pretty farty.	Simethicone (Gas-X, Mylanta Gas) is safe.	The gas must pass, so you don't have to bring it up. You may have to suffer through that farty bedroom for awhile, caveman.
What if she has diarrhea or constipation?	Loperamide (Imodium AD) for diarrhea is OK as directed. Fiber laxatives (Metamucil, Benefiber, Citrucel) for constipation is good.	Diarrhea for more than a few days may cause dehydration, so call the doc if it persists. Fruit and vegetables and plenty of H_2O can help things to get moving.
What about hemorrhoids?	Try witch hazel (Tucks Pads) or hydrocortisone (Anusol HC). Both are completely safe as directed.	Again, a well-balanced diet with light exercise may help. Sitting for too long can make things worse.
Vaginal yeast infection?	Some safe topical medications include clotrimazole (Monistat), miconazole (Gyne-Lotrimin) and butoconazole (Femstat).	If untreated, a "down-there" infection can cause some problems, so if meds don't seem to help, call the OB-GYN.

DR. BRIAN

HERBAL REMEDIES: THE KIND AND THE UNKIND

Just because it's deemed natural, nonsynthetic, homeopathic, or herbal, and it's found in a health food store doesn't mean it's safe for an expectant mom to ingest. While many herbs offer benefits and are not generally considered toxic, a lack of research and government oversight with some of them suggests that an expectant mom use caution and consult her doctor before taking herbal nutritional supplements and other homeopathic medicines. Generally speaking, doctors suggest that women don't use them the first trimester, and if they do use them later in pregnancy, to do so in lower doses for shorter intervals.

Herbs that **SHOULD BE AVOIDED** in pregnancy include:

- ▶ **FEVERFEW** (used for migraines; may cause uterine contractions)

- ▶ **GINSENG** (may cause uterine contractions);

- ▶ **GOLDENSEAL** (may cause uterine contractions)

- ▶ **KAVA KAVA** (used for anxiety; may cause fetal sedation)

Herbs generally **CONSIDERED SAFE** include:

- ▶ **ECHINACEA**
- ▶ **GINKGO BILOBA**
- ▶ **ST. JOHN'S WORT**
- ▶ **MILK THISTLE**
- ▶ **VALERIAN**

CATEGORY C: Evidence of adverse effects on fetus in animal studies; the drug should be given only if potential benefits of doing so outweigh potential risks to the fetus.

CATEGORY D: Positive evidence of human fetal risk, but the benefits from use may outweigh the risks.

CATEGORY X: Studies in animals or humans show direct link to fetal abnormalities or fetal risk; that risk outweighs any possible benefit, so women who are or may become pregnant should not use the drug.

Most prescription medications fall into either the B or C category because of a lack of studies on human subjects. Thus, many B and C drugs are considered safe for pregnant women. The risk associated with specific medications tends to fluctuate according to what stage of pregnancy a woman is in. But generally speaking, the following are several of the most common prescription meds considered teratogenic (toxic) to expectant mom and/or fetus:

- ▶ **ANTI-CONVULSANTS** (seizure prevention drugs)

- ▶ **ANDROGENS** (a type of hormone)

- ▶ **DANAZOLE** (used to treat endometriosis, fibrocystic breast disease, etc.)

- ▶ **RETINOIDS** (like Accutane, used to treat severe acne)

- ▶ **LITHIUM** (for bipolar disorder)

OLDER AND WISER

Here's to you, Mrs. Robinson...
—SIMON & GARFUNKEL

If age was expressed in terms of mental and emotional development, the caveman would be stuck in his infancy and any female with whom he coupled would be an "older woman," regardless of her physical age relative to his.

For the most part, however, we still rely on the calendar to measure age. And these days, more "older women" are having children well into their thirties and even in their forties. Pregnancy for women thirty-five and older raises special medical issues. In the first place, it can be tougher for women of that age to conceive, since their fertility level tends to erode gradually after age thirty. And once a thirty-five-plus-year-old woman does get pregnant, there are other considerations.

➤ They are more apt to have preexisting illnesses that could affect health during pregnancy.

➤ They face a higher risk of pregnancy-related complications, like high blood pressure, diabetes, and placenta previa.

➤ They have an increased chance of having a baby with a genetic disorder such as Down syndrome.

These potentialities increase the likelihood she will be subjected to more medical tests, such as amniocentesis, when pregnant. Older pregnant women also may be subject to more interventions in labor and delivery, including monitoring, anesthesia, and an increased chance of cesarean section. There's also a higher rate of unexplained sudden fetal death late in pregnancy (one in 440 as opposed to one in a thousand for younger women).

It's not all bad news, however. Besides being more seasoned lovers and more experienced life companions, older women may:

➤ Be more secure economically

➤ Be better equipped to make wise decisions about pregnancy

➤ Have better people skills and confidence to ask for what they need

➤ Be healthier than their twentysomething counterparts, with a lifestyle more conducive to childbearing and childrearing

Bottom line: while having a baby after thirty-five may be slightly riskier for a woman, the likelihood of having a healthy pregnancy and offspring is still very strong.

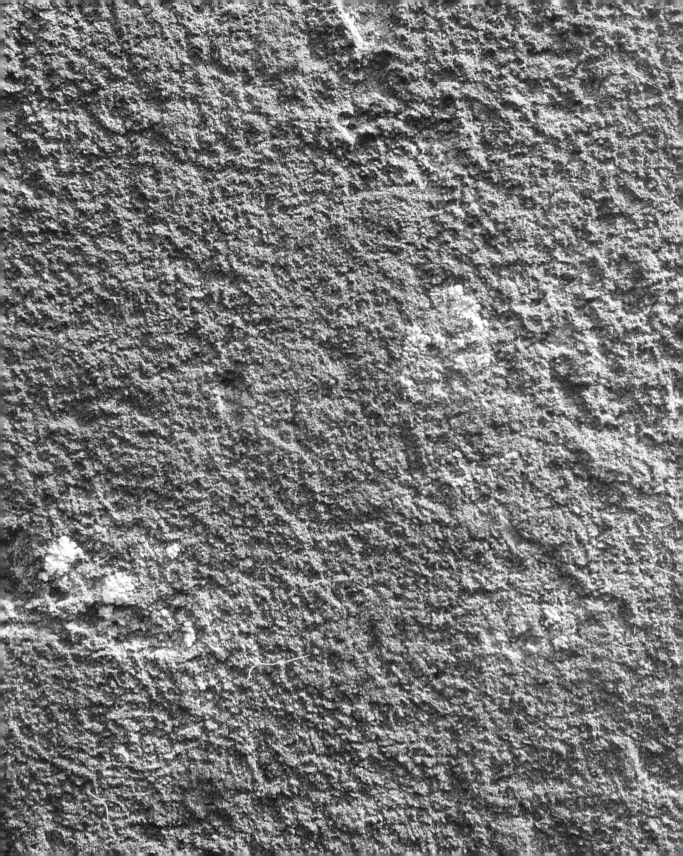

CHAPTER 5

JUST THE TWO OF US

*It's the end of the world as we know it
And I feel fine.*

—R.E.M.

IT'S FOUR A.M. in Las Vegas and four men sit facing the dealer, the sole combatants at the only open $5 blackjack table in this dank downtown casino. Gronk and his bachelor buddies are in Sin City for a weekend dedicated to scratching some of their primal (and if his buddies get their way, illegal) caveman urges and sending Gronk, the expectant father, off into parenthood with a bang.

The men, each looking slightly unkempt and unfocused, exchange few words as chips change hands. After a run of especially poor hands, punctuated by the dealer nailing twenty-ones on three consecutive hands, one of Gronk's friends leans over to offer some unsolicited advice.

"Have you ever considered that this trip could be the end, the last hurrah for the four of us? You have a kid on the way. You're done, dude. Life is over. We'll never see you on a Vegas trip again. Nice knowing you."

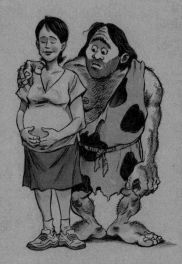

GROW WITH GRONK

What the caveman stands to gain from reading Chapter 5:

▶ **THE ABILITY** to discern between solid and suspect advice for expectant parents

▶ **STRATEGIES** for the expectant couple to enjoy pregnancy to its fullest

▶ **INSIGHT** into the pregnant woman's mind

▶ **THE KNOW-HOW** to preserve a solid, if sometimes sporadic, sex life during pregnancy

▶ **AN UNDERSTANDING** of the benefits of attending a birthing or parenting class

▶ **THE IMPETUS** to start an exercise program tailored to both caveman and pregnant woman

The conversation ends as the friend hits on a seventeen looking at the dealer's six. His statement lingers in the air, however. It's the first time Gronk hears someone analyze his pending parenthood situation in such a primitive manner. But it certainly won't be the last. As expectant parents, one thing you and your woman will never want for is advice. Some you may welcome. But a vast volume of it will come uninvited from people who feel compelled to tell you exactly what's going to happen to you, when and why it's going to happen, and how you and your woman should deal with it. (Admittedly, the content of this book falls into that category.) With so much information bombarding the two of you from so many different angles, how is the couple to distinguish between sound, valid advice, well meaning but misguided wisdom, and unadulterated bluster? For a guy who's not espe-

cially adept at filtering and processing vast amounts of information, this can be a frustrating undertaking.

It helps to consider the source. Put too much stock in advice provided by "reliable sources" in the locker room, at poker games, tailgate parties, and on the barstool next to you, for instance, and you soon may

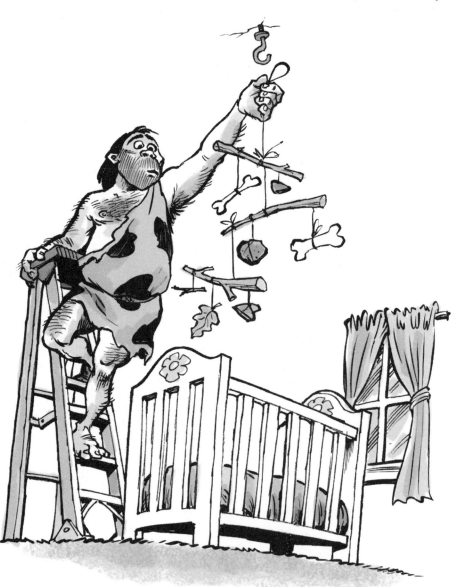

find yourself utterly confused. Pregnancy, they contend, marks the beginning of the end—the end of an active social life, the end of a regular workout regimen, the end of eating out, playing golf, taking vacations, napping, and enjoying time to yourself; in a nutshell, the end of independence. But this widely held view is not only unenlightened, it's inaccurate.

Granted, becoming an expectant parent marks passage into unfamiliar territory and an important new stage of life. With pregnancy and then a new baby, major life changes are inevitable. You will have less free time and more responsibility. However, contrary to the picture your caveman comrades may paint for you in the shadowy recesses of smoky poker rooms and sweaty locker rooms, a positive pregnancy test doesn't mean the end of life as you and your woman know it. In fact, that picture, perpetuated by generations of cavemen before you, is fraught with misconception, fallacy, and outright delusion.

Life as you know it will *not* end at pregnancy and childbirth if you don't let it. No doubt, the dynamics of your life will change to some extent. You still control your own destiny, however, although to a lesser extent than you did before (remember, the me-first stage of your life has passed).

Remember, too, that during pregnancy the two of you still get to enjoy many of the things that made you a solid couple in the first place—taking the dog for a hike, traveling, working out together, hanging out with friends, sharing intimate moments, going to dinner and a movie, roasting a freshly killed boar over an open pit, whatever floats your boat. What's more, since you are now expecting, the pregnancy frontier provides new opportunities to add dimension to your relationship, from doing projects together around the home to shopping for baby gear to inventing and exploring new sexual positions to accommodate your woman's shifting center of gravity.

The stress and anxiety that come with pending parenthood can divide expectant parents at exactly the time they should be drawing closer and celebrating the offspring their union will soon bring. During a time when you're both dealing with baby-related angst and apprehension, you can serve as one another's tonic by making a point of spending quality time together, having fun as a couple, and savoring the last months of childlessness.

Stress relief for pregnant couples comes in a variety of forms. Most importantly, don't deny one another time to yourselves. When you're busy and tense, sometimes the best antidote is to spend time alone reading a good book, going for a run, napping, listening to music, or simply vegetating in front of the television.

As important as alone time is to your psyche, pregnancy is no time to neglect your partner. Quite the opposite. Your mission is to prove that, contrary to the uninformed assertions of your Cro-Magnon cronies, an expectant couple can have a life that doesn't revolve exclusively around that bun in the oven. It's all the better if the two of you can keep the fire stoked while also building mental and physical strength and breaking new ground in your relationship. Here are a few proven methods for preserving and even improving your quality of life during pregnancy:

▶ **EXERCISE TOGETHER.** Starting and sticking to a regular workout routine benefits man, woman, and gestating caveling.

▶ **PRESERVE INTIMACY** and at least occasionally fulfill one another's sexual urges. Sex is the engine of the human species. But sometimes during pregnancy the engine's spark plugs fail to fire. As a couple, it's often fun, sometimes challenging, and usually worthwhile to explore ways of keeping the spark alive.

▶ **SHARE WHAT'S ON YOUR MIND.** It's not always easy for the caveman to communicate his thoughts, emotions, fears, and aspirations, even with the person he is most intimate with. Make a point of keeping the lines of communication open. Guys who bottle up their feelings can become ticking time bombs, ready to explode.

▶ **SHARE YOUR VISIONS** of how your lives might unfold going forward: finances, to work or not to work while raising a child, to have more children, etc. The less frequently you discuss major issues like this, generally the more pressure you're likely to feel as the baby's birth draws closer.

▶ **REVEL IN THE NESTING INSTINCT,** which provides the nervous energy you need to complete every home project un-

der the sun, from decorating the nursery to seeding the lawn and beyond.

▶ **TAKE SOME FORM OF BIRTHING OR PARENTAL PREP CLASS.** The more prepared the two of you are for labor, childbirth, and early parenthood, the less freaked out you likely will be when her water breaks and the contractions begin. These classes also can connect you with other expectant couples with whom you can compare notes and develop friendships.

Something else for the prehistoric pupil to keep in mind: while these classes can be a little too touchy-feely for your tastes, you score big points with your mate merely for being present and engaging yourself in class activities. As with the SATs, you get credit for simply showing up with your pencil.

▶ **TOSS AROUND NAME IDEAS.** Mix legitimate names with ridiculous or homemade ones (Brundt, Grout, Bilda, Cumulous) during the conversation to keep things loose.

▶ **TAKE A BREAK.** Plan one or two weekend getaways. The first you can take around the beginning of the second trimester, when your woman's bouts with nausea are abating and blood-flow to her genitals is robust. The second can happen sometime later in the second trimester or early in the third—but not so late that she won't be able to fully enjoy the excursion or won't be able to go because her doctor recommends she not travel.

LOST IN TRANSLATION

As a modern missing link for whom nuance and shading are foreign concepts, reading between the lines isn't one of your strong suits. You may spend a ton of time with your woman, yet still not be perceptive enough to tell when what she says isn't necessarily what she means.

Especially during pregnancy, the ability to glean hidden meaning from your woman's words becomes an important, necessary skill for a man to have. She wants to send you some sort of message but doesn't want to come right out and say it. She may be: (a) testing you to see if you're listening—*really listening*—to her, (b) tired of having to explicitly spell *everything* out to you in the plainest English, or (c) like many pregnant women, feeling a bit too scatterbrained to actually piece together the words necessary to get her point across.

The caveman who repeatedly fails to extract the true meaning of his woman's words will face the wrath of a pregnant partner who has lost her patience because she believes her man misunderstands or misinterprets her. On the other hand, the guy who develops skills as a translator earns the right to be called a "good communicator," a man who genuinely understands the female perspective.

To develop those skills a man has to be able to climb inside a woman's head and actually *think* like a woman. That ability doesn't come overnight for the caveman, who has enough difficulty thinking like a modern man, never mind a modern woman. During the learning process, you will occasionally misinterpret or miss altogether the signals she's sending you. When she asks you to go rent a movie, for example, you may assume she wants you to bring home *Scarface, Reservoir Dogs, Predator* or *Caddyshack* when instead you should be thinking more along the lines of *Gone With the Wind, Boys on the Side, Terms of Endearment* or anything with Brad Pitt wearing pelts and riding a horse.

Here are examples of how an expectant Gronk put his skills as a listener and interpreter to good use. Keep in mind, responses must be delivered with sincerity. Insincerity—sideways grin, lack of eye contact, fidgeting—will be detected and construed as groveling, rendering your response inappropriate.

SHE SAYS	SHE MEANS
I can't find anything to wear. None of my clothes fit.	*I feel fat and unattractive.*
Are you excited for my mom to come?	*You are going to be seeing a lot of your mother-in-law, so adjust and be on your best behavior.*
My bras don't fit anymore.	*My God, my breasts are larger than they've ever been and they hurt.*
This place is a wreck and I'm tired.	*You might consider lifting a finger to clean and maintain our home.*
Why don't you call so-and-so and go play thirty-six holes?	*Give me a few hours to myself, starting right now.*
You're going out to play golf again?	*I feel as if I'm going through this pregnancy alone.*
What do you want to do for dinner?	*I don't care how you do it, just see to it that there's a meal in front of me within thirty minutes.*
My back/my feet are sore.	*Get over here and rub me—and do apply the massage techniques you learned earlier in the book you're reading.*
Are you *really* going out with the boys tonight?	*I'm feeling a little insecure and don't want you out at a bar with your single friends, with single women lurking.*
We need to organize the garage, build more shelves, and sweep the crawl space.	*There's a baby coming, but we're not prepared and neither is our home.*
I haven't felt the baby move this week, so I set up a doctor's appointment. You don't really need to come with me, Gronk.	*I'm freaking out because I haven't felt the baby move much lately. Drop what you're doing and come with me to the doctor's.*
I'm feeling a little overwhelmed.	*I need a hug.*

THE UNCULTIVATED RESPONSE	GRONK'S ACTUAL RESPONSE
ALL WOMEN GET LARGE WHEN THEY'RE PREGNANT. WHAT DID YOU EXPECT?	*He buys a gift certificate at a clothing store, provides flowery but not overtly pandering compliments about his woman's beauty and radiance*
EXACTLY HOW LONG WILL SHE BE STAYING?	*Upon mother-in-law's arrival, he treats the two of them to a day at the spa and an evening out to dinner.*
SURE, THEY'RE GREAT NOW. BUT WHAT HAPPENS TO THEM IN FIVE YEARS?	*"Let's adjourn to the bedroom," he says. "I'm getting turned on."*
I'VE GOT THIS NAGGING BACK THING. WHAT I NEED IS REST.	*He gets to it or enlists some help by securing a cleaning service. It makes everyone's life much easier.*
NO, I THINK I'M GOING TO ROOST HERE ON THE COUCH AND WATCH THE GAME.	*He hits 'em long and straight, goes low, and most of all, enjoys himself, because it could be his last round for a while.*
IF I DON'T PLAY TODAY, HOW'S MY SHORT GAME EVER GOING TO GET BETTER?	*He says, "You know, there are a few projects I could be doing around here."*
YOU GO AHEAD AND FEND FOR YOURSELF, HONEY. I ALREADY ATE.	*He checks the fridge for the right ingredients to make a quick meal based on a recipe from Chapter 6. If that's not an option, he turns to leftovers or take-out/delivery.*
MAYBE YOU SHOULD TRY A DIFFERENT PAIR OF SHOES.	*He lights some candles, puts on some mood music, dons his masseur outfit and starts rubbing.*
YEP, THEY THINK BEING WITH AN EXPECTANT FATHER MAKES THE CHICKS TAKE THEM MORE SERIOUSLY.	*He reassures her she's more beautiful than ever, then goes out with his friends. But he makes a point of coming home earlier than she expects so he has time to dispense a foot rub before bedtime.*
LET YOUR PARENTS TAKE CARE OF THAT STUFF WHEN THEY GET HERE.	*He spearheads a clean-and-purge effort. He jettisons the vintage Molly Hatchet concert T-shirt and the wooden golf clubs.*
THAT'S INTERESTING. GIVE ME A CALL ONCE THE APPOINTMENT IS OVER TO LET ME KNOW WHAT THE DOCTOR SAYS.	*He joins her for this doctor's appointment and as many others as he can, especially if she seems nervous.*
THERE'S NOTHING TO FEEL OVERWHELMED ABOUT. WE'LL BE FINE ONCE THIS IS OVER.	*He provides a long, heartfelt embrace, cooks her dinner, then offers a massage to release some of her stress.*

THE CAVA SUTRA: SEX AND THE EXPECTANT COUPLE

*I'm primitive, I'm a primitive man
I got a primitive girl, we make
    primitive love
I'm a Stone Age Romeo, I got a
    space-age Juliet
We make primitive love, 'cause I ain't
    got a TV set*

—HOODOO GURUS,
"MARS NEEDS GUITARS"

*In order to seduce a woman, it is necessary
to know erotic technique....For erotic
success, the peculiarities of both parties
must be known before commencing
to embrace. Skill is required to cause
excitation.*

—THE COMPLETE KAMA SUTRA,
TRANSLATED BY ALAIN DANIÉLOU

Achieving the "erotic success" to which Indian sexpert Vatsyayana referred some 1,700 years ago in his ancient but still relevant lovemaking textbook, the *Kama Sutra*, can be a tall task during pregnancy. From the Stone Age Romeo's perspective, techniques that have worked wonders on a woman in the past may not push the right buttons now. This may prompt an amorous but confounded Cro-Magnon lover to question his own manhood and wonder whether his skills and ability to please are diminishing.

You're still a relatively young guy, so diminished skills and a lack of manhood probably aren't the cause. More likely the root of the problem is a misunderstanding of what Vatsyayana referred to as the "peculiarities of both parties." Pregnancy manifests a range of unusual and unexpected physical and mental changes, some of which can have a major bearing on a couple's sex life. As Vatsyayana—who quite obviously was a cultivated caveman in his own right—so succinctly points out, "Skill

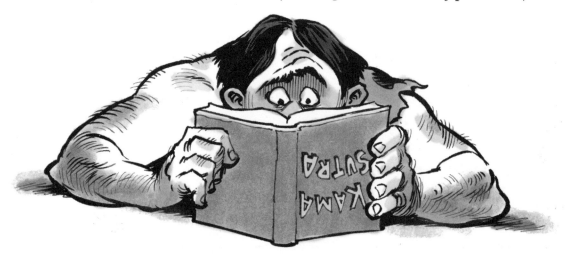

THE AGONY AND THE ECSTASY: WHAT'S SHAPING YOUR SEX LIFE?

FRISKY BUSINESS: FACTORS THAT GET THE JUICES FLOWING

I am woman, you are man I am gentle so you can be barbarian

—THE SUPREMES, "I AM WOMAN"

MENTAL FACTORS	♂	♀	PHYSICAL FACTORS	♂	♀
Accustomed to regular sexual activity	X	X	Energy restored as hormone levels return to balance		X
Aroused by partner's fuller breasts	X		Increased blood flow to genitals		X
Curious about making love with pregnant woman and trying new sexual positions necessitated by pregnancy	X		Increased vaginal lubrication		X
Free of contraception concerns	X	X	Fuller breasts		X
Desire to maintain intimacy with and please partner	X	X	Need to release tension, stress	X	X

NO CAN DO: COMMON REASONS FOR THE COLD SHOULDER

I hear you knocking but you can't come in

—DAVE EDMUNDS, "I HEAR YOU KNOCKING"

MENTAL FACTORS	♂	♀	PHYSICAL FACTORS	♂	♀
Anxiety, fears associated with pending parenthood	X	X	General fatigue, pain, discomfort		X
General loss of libido	X	X	Doctor's orders/medical condition		X
Fear of hurting baby	X	X	Nausea caused by increased estrogen level (especially during first trimester)		X
Couvade (see p. 24)	X		Physical awkwardness		X
Worried it will be painful		X	Mood swings caused by hormonal changes		X
Insecurity about pregnant body		X	Tender breasts		X
Mood swings	X	X	Hemorrhoids		X
Feeling neglected, "left out"	X				
In-laws/parents sleeping in the bedroom next door	X	X			

DR. BRIAN

HOW TO PUT A REALLY PREGNANT PARTNER "OVER THE HUMP"

Sex may be the furthest thing from your mind as your baby's due date approaches. But in cases where the woman's body is ready for labor and all she wants is to deliver the package and put an end to her discomfort, sexual intercourse may be just what she needs to push her closer to the delivery room. That's because of a hormone called prostaglandin, which is found in a male's semen and has a softening effect on a woman's cervix. Although a guy's body (even a caveguy's) cannot supply enough of the hormone to single-handedly cause preterm labor, he can supply enough to get the process moving when the woman's body and the baby are ready. It's also been shown that when a woman has an orgasm or her nipples are stimulated, her body produces a chemical called oxytocin, which may help trigger contractions at full term. So when her patience has worn thin and she feels ready to pop, sex may be the last thing on her mind but exactly what her body ordered. If she summons you to the bedroom, it's time to punch in for a little overtime duty.

is required to cause excitation"; having the prowess to arouse and please a pregnant woman demands that the caveman adjust his techniques to accommodate the peculiarities that may come with carrying a child in one's womb.

Some couples may find that their sexual urges and activity continue unabated during pregnancy. The most fortunate twosomes may even experience an increase in their coital urges. Others may see their desires diminish. At times one or both of you will feel "too pooped to pop." Depending on how active your sex life was prior to conception, this can be a new phenomenon or familiar territory. Whatever was the case, given how preoccupied both of you are with wrapping your minds around the changes you are confronting, there will be moments when neither of you may feel like wrapping your arms and legs around one another. No words need be exchanged; you'll look one another in the eye and know now's not the time, then silently seal the evening's vow of celibacy by returning to your respective sides of the bed and burying your nose in the book (or men's magazine) you are reading.

You've lost that lovin' feeling
Oh, oh, that lovin' feeling
You've lost that lovin' feeling
Now it's gone, gone, gone, oh, oh, oh.

—THE RIGHTEOUS BROTHERS,
"YOU'VE LOST THAT LOVIN' FEELING"

A lack of sexual desire is nothing to be especially concerned about, unless the malaise persists for weeks on end. If you or your woman find yourselves taking cold showers to keep your blood from boiling due to sexual inactivity, it's time to find a means of releasing the tension. You can surmise what that means: sometimes you may need to be your own best friend.

Indeed, it's not unusual during pregnancy for one person to be in the mood for love and the other to be in the mood for slumber. Diminished sexual desire during pregnancy is fairly common — and contrary to what you've heard or assume, the woman isn't always the one with the limp libido. Guys can experience a drop-off in their sexual urges as well.

It can be difficult to pinpoint what causes reduced sex drive during pregnancy, but a variety of mental and physical factors can contribute to the condition, as specified in the "Agony and Ecstasy" grid (see p. 97). In many cases a lack of sex drive can be attributed to more than one factor.

Hormonal changes are one of the factors that shape a childbearing woman's sexual appetite. In some women a change in hormonal levels can cause a surge in sexual drives; with others it has the opposite effect. In many cases hormones can increase a woman's friskiness at some points during pregnancy and curb her carnal appetite at other points. Fluctuations in a woman's sexual urges — and thus the fate of a couple's sex life in general — also can be linked directly to any discomfort she's experiencing as her bodily proportions change. She is likely to feel less limber, more awkward, and

DR. BRIAN

YOUR WEAPON IS NO THREAT TO THE BABY

You're proud of your manhood, but when confronted with the idea of sex during pregnancy, a question comes to mind that paralyzes you with concern: can a man's sex organ possibly hurt a fetus? Good question, but one prompted more by misconception and urban legend than truth. In fact, the baby is very well protected in the womb. For women who are deemed to be having a healthy or "normal" pregnancy, prenatal sex does not harm the fetus. During intercourse the mucus plug (located in the cervix), amniotic sac, and the musculature of the uterus prevent the penis from contacting the baby. So be proud of your manhood, but don't worry about it causing damage.

more self-conscious about her appearance—conditions that are not especially conducive to uninhibited lovemaking.

It is next to impossible to predict exactly how the dynamics of your sex life will change when you're expecting; each couple's experience during pregnancy is different. While that makes trend-spotting difficult, many couples plot a common course on the sexual activity curve: the frequency of their sexual interludes drops off during the first trimester, largely because of nausea and the newness of the situation, rebounds somewhat during the second trimester as hormone levels stabilize and the mind acclimates to the pregnancy concept, only to drop again in the third trimester as her discomfort level increases and baby thoughts (in both of you) overshadow primal sexual urges. There may be a flurry of sexual activity as she approaches and reaches term, when (as Dr. Brian points out) it has been shown that intercourse and other hanky-panky can jumpstart labor.

The swirling cauldron of hormonal and mental upheaval during pregnancy can make for some unfamiliar and vexing bedroom dynamics for the expectant couple. Here are some of the questions that arise:

- At what points during pregnancy is a woman more and less likely to feel frisky?

- How about a man—under what conditions is he more or less apt to yearn for hanky-panky?

- When one person wants it but the other doesn't, how do you bridge the gap?

- When the fact that neither person has wanted it for a while becomes an issue, how does the couple rekindle the flame?

- When both want it all the time, how do they find the time, the energy, and the right position?

When, for whatever reason, sex is out of the question for one or both of you, there's no point in pushing the matter. Do what Gronk did during the dry spells of pregnancy: go out and run six or eight miles, shirtless, in forty-degree weather. But where there is a will to have sex, there is a way, even during the third trimester when, mentally, you are both feeling the heat of pending parenthood, and physically, your woman is at her most uncomfortable and awkward.

Those formidable obstacles can be overcome if your sexual urges or desire for intimacy is strong enough. When you and your woman have exchanged the telltale eyebrow raise that says it's time to scratch the primal itch, yet you somehow still can't seem to conjure the mental or physical drive necessary, here are a few suggestions for tapping that elusive reserve of latent sexual energy:

- **MASSAGE:** Touch leads to intimacy, which in turn can lead to lovemaking.

- **BATHING TOGETHER:** Something about water gets people wet.

- **ROMANCE:** In wintertime, take the well-tested route of cooking her a gourmet dinner, then retiring to the den, where you've lit a fire in the fireplace, put on some soulful mood music, and rolled out an animal pelt (imitation or the skin of your own captured quarry) from your "collection."

▶ **MOVIES AND MAGAZINES:** Visual stimulation works well for some couples. Here's a good chance for the caveman to make constructive use of another of his hitherto hidden "collections." (Friends may be happy to donate a few items from their collections to the cause.)

▶ **SNUGGLING:** Caveman may want to cut right to the chase. But females often prefer a more less-deliberate approach and may need to be coaxed with light contact through spooning, hugging, and the like.

Now you're both in the mood. There's no time to waste, lest one of you lose that loving feeling. But wait! Before you lumber into the familiar, reliable missionary position, you need to consider your woman's shifting physical dimensions. The missionary position becomes difficult, then next to impossible as her abdomen grows. There also are medical considerations associated with the old standby guy-on-top position. Beginning early in the second trimester, doctors tend to discourage pregnant women from supine exercise. And the missionary position is exactly that kind of exercise, at least if the activity lasts more than a few fleeting moments. At about the fourth month of pregnancy, the weight of the baby begins exerting more pressure on the expectant mom's aorta. This can decrease blood flow to her uterine artery, the main source of oxygen to the placenta, which nourishes the gestat-

ing caveling. Lying in a supine position also can hamper the return of blood to the pregnant woman's heart.

With the missionary position thus no longer an option, now is your opportunity for adventure. Here's a chance to tap your latent caveman sexual instincts by trying different sexual maneuvers and perhaps even inventing a new one. For additional ideas, secure a copy of the *Kama Sutra* (preferably an illustrated version), in which our kindred caveman spirit Vatsyayana provides compelling, methodical details on "the thirteen methods of sexual penetration." At least a few of those may come in handy when things between you and your woman get hot and heavy. Here are several worth exploring, if you haven't already:

▶ **WOMAN ON TOP:** When the guy is on the bottom, he bears much of the weight of her pregnant belly, not the woman. Not that he particularly minds a little extra weight anyway. There are several spins on this position. One has the man with his legs extended flat, his arms propping his torso up, with the woman on his lap, her legs spread. Another has the woman sitting astride him, supporting herself with her arms, while he lies on the bed.

▶ **SIDE-BY-SIDE (SIDE-LYING):** This position can be approached in either of two ways—facing one another or man behind woman. In the Kama Sutra, the face-to-face position is called the "lateral box" or parshva samputa. The

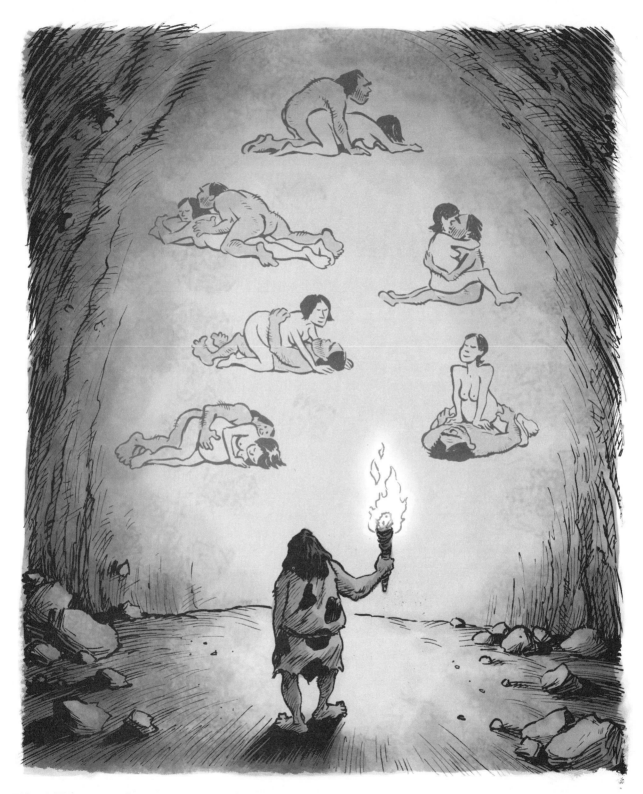

side-by-side, back-to-front position is sometimes called the "spoon position."

▶ **MAN BEHIND:** The main copulative position for generations of cavemen, this technique now is popularly known as "doggy style"—no more need be said.

▶ **THE LEAPFROG:** The woman kneels with legs spread. She leans forward, using her arms for support as the man approaches from behind.

▶ **THE SPREAD EAGLE:** Another rear-entry position—this one most suitable for early pregnancy, before the size of her belly precludes such activity—it is achieved when the woman lies face down, the caveman on top of her, supporting his weight with his arms. She spreads her legs and—voila!

▶ **SIT, BOY, SIT:** Here's one that requires a prop—any chair will suffice; one with a cushioned seat to soften the impact on the caveman's bottom. The guy sits in the chair facing forward while his partner sits on his lap, facing him. It's also worth trying this position with the woman similarly astride him on his lap but with her back to him.

▶ **POSITIONS TO ASK YOUR DOCTOR ABOUT BEFORE ATTEMPTING, DURING PREGNANCY AND OTHERWISE:** the Wheelbarrow, the Cuban Missile Crisis, the Broken Flute.

DR. BRIAN

WHEN IT'S TOO RISKY TO GET FRISKY

The doctor just uttered the words you hoped you'd never hear: **ABSOLUTELY NO INTERCOURSE.** Women who are diagnosed with any of a number of conditions may be advised to cease having intercourse because it could put her health and that of the fetus at risk. Any of the following conditions could prompt your woman's doctor to put prenatal sex on hold, at least temporarily:

▶ If she is diagnosed with placenta previa, a condition in which the placenta is covering all or part of the cervix

▶ If she has previously had preterm labor or birth

▶ If she has had more than one miscarriage

▶ If she exhibits symptoms such as cramping or contractions that indicate a preterm labor is possible

▶ If she has vaginal bleeding

▶ If she is leaking amniotic fluid (the fluid in the sac surrounding the baby)

▶ If she contracts an infection

▶ If she has a cervical condition that raises her risk of miscarriage or premature delivery

If your partner believes she has any of the above conditions, have her see her doctor before your next roll in the hay.

PONDER THIS

THE NESTING INSTINCT

Why is your woman spending so much time arranging and rearranging the baby clothes? What's the source of your strange and persistent urge to stockpile a year's supply of canned goods in the basement? You have heard of the phenomenon, and here in pregnancy, you and your woman are experiencing it firsthand: the nesting instinct. In the name of making one's surroundings safe, organized, and comfortable, manifested as a primal, urgent drive to complete home projects and tie up every one of life's loose ends, you begin shoring up your nest in anticipation of the baby's arrival home.

Common among expectant men and women, nesting urges in humans are instinctive behaviors akin to rodents shredding newspaper into small bits and making a nest of them to house their young. Some people feel these urges acutely, others not at all. A person who has them generally feels compelled to put one's house in order before the baby is born. This behavior makes sense: take care of the things you need to take care of now, because once you have a child, you will have even less time to get it all done. You know, things like purging the basement, cleaning out the crawl space, painstakingly organizing dresser drawers with three years' worth of infant and toddler clothing, and establishing a rigid schedule for family and friends to visit the newborn.

Keep in mind, the less you resist the nesting instinct, the more you can channel the energy it generates toward constructive purposes. Finally you will find the energy reserve needed to finish painting the nursery at two a.m. on a Tuesday.

WE DON'T NEED NO EDUCATION— OR DO WE?

Through childhood, your school years, and now in your adult life, you have managed to muddle through the many academic, social, domestic, and professional challenges thrown at you by relying almost exclusively on your caveman instincts. You've used your intellect to supplement your gut when absolutely necessary—to pass a test on which securing your diploma depended, to impress a woman you coveted, or to provide your boss with a solid argument for giving you a salary bump.

Now your woman's pregnancy confronts you with weighty questions you cannot answer instinctively or intuitively. What exactly will your role and responsibilities be during the birthing process? How to explain what's happening to your partner physically and mentally? How does something that size fit through an opening that small? How does one avoid passing out when viewing such anatomically graphic and intensely sanguine sights?

For many expectant parents, the answers to these and other pregnancy and childbirth questions will be revealed only with help and input from others more experienced in the field than you. That's right, Mr. Prehistoric Pupil, it may be time for you to return to the classroom—with or without your partner—to prepare yourself for pregnancy, childbirth, and parenting. Relying on an expert's wisdom and guidance in preparing for the potentially arduous journey that lies ahead is by no means an admission of failure. In fact, even the most evolved members of the human race can sometimes find themselves lost in the pregnancy and childbirth wilderness, especially if they are first-time parents.

There are many compelling reasons for expectant moms and dads to go back to class. For a minimal commitment of time and money, expectant parents can learn about the physical, physiological, and mental aspects of pregnancy, how a woman's labor and delivery might unfold, relaxation techniques to use during labor, plus practicalities such as how to change a diaper, bathe an infant, and put a baby in a car seat. There's also the chance to meet, compare notes, and bond with classmates who are in the same boat as you. This lays the groundwork for potential social interaction between your children once they are born. (Note to caveman: back in the Stone Age, expectant parents may have used this type of setting to arrange marriages between their unborn children; given how our society has evolved, such preordained unions are no longer considered appropriate or acceptable.)

Many a male has been overwhelmed during labor and delivery because he wasn't prepared for what he encountered. A majority of guys who graduated from some sort of prenatal class will attest that the stuff they learned there made them better equipped and more confident in their ability to tackle the rigors of bringing a baby into the world.

Just knowing that other guys are going through precisely the same thing at roughly the same time as you is reassuring.

These days expectant parents have access to a wide variety of preparatory classes designed specifically for dads-to-be and moms-to-be individually and as a couple. Typically offered by hospitals, birthing centers, health groups, and community organizations, classes can range from multiweek to partial-day prep courses. There are birthing and early parenting classes for couples, boot camps for expectant fathers, and breast-feeding courses for expectant mothers. Classes may be offered to groups or privately to individual couples. Most expectant parents who chose to supplement their instincts with pregnancy and childbirth classwork will tell you it was a valuable experience. In doing so, you have little to lose and much to gain. What's more, these typically are classes for which Stone Age students cannot receive a failing grade. You will have little or no homework. Your teacher will not call you out for nose picking during class.

Even if you choose not to take a class prior to the birth of your child, at minimum you should consider touring the facility where you plan to have the birth so you have a feel for the place whose halls you likely will be pacing before, during, and after delivery.

FIT FOR PARENTHOOD

We gotta get out while we're young
'Cause tramps like us, baby, we were
born to run

—BRUCE SPRINGSTEEN, "BORN TO RUN"

Obesity is rampant in America. Here in the twenty-first century we are eating less healthy food in larger quantities while doing less to burn off at least some of what we consume. As a society we're generally a bunch of doughboys and doughgirls with no business wearing spandex clothing as often as we do. Between 1980 and 2000, obesity rates doubled among adults. According to the Centers for Disease Control and Prevention, roughly sixty million adults—a whopping 30 percent of the adult population here in the United States—are obese. Obesity can lead to such serious conditions as diabetes, heart disease, cancer, and arthritis, while being overweight as an adult may cause high blood pressure and increase cholesterol levels.

We haven't always had a problem with flab. Back in prehistoric times, long before spandex was invented, people spent much of their time on such physically demanding, calorie-burning pursuits as stalking prey, climbing trees to gather nuts, and bludgeoning members of a rival clan with clubs. Obesity and inactivity were not issues. Indeed, people's life spans were so short they didn't have time to pack on the pounds. Walking, running, and vine-swinging were the cavedweller's sole means of propulsion; meanwhile, nuts and berries, not junk food, were a large part of the prehistoric diet.

But here in the era of cars, computers, remote-control devices, supersize meals, and leather recliners, we're spending more time in repose and less time being physically active. The results are obvious to behold. We're less fit and less inclined to do anything about it.

But just because you and your woman are expecting a baby doesn't mean you have to turn into slugs and resign yourselves to membership in the Overstuffed Underexercised Club. In fact, being physically fit could make you generally more fit to handle pregnancy, childbirth, and parenting. Here again you have a chance not only to do something as a couple that's good for both of you in the short term, but also to introduce a routine that can be a positive force in your lives for decades to come. Seize the opportunity now to develop a fitness routine and you will be developing healthy habits that can take pounds off your frame, make you stronger and more resilient (so you can better cope with reduced and interrupted sleep), and actually extend your lifespan.

Wait until the baby is born to get in shape and you may find you have neither the energy nor the time to start a fitness routine. But if you enter parenthood with a regular workout routine in place, you put yourself in an excellent position to sustain at least some semblance of that routine once the baby is born.

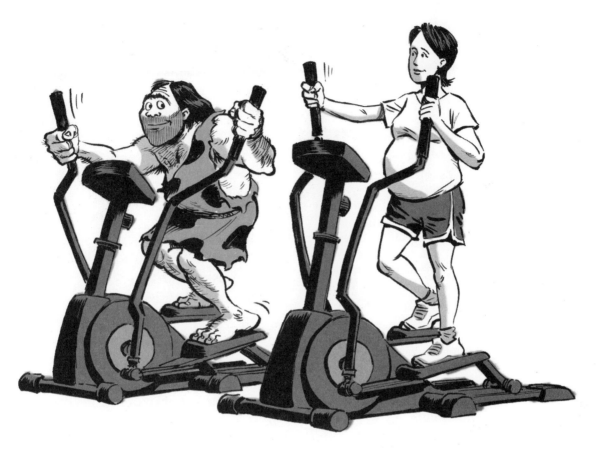

If you exercise regularly, you likely already know some of the benefits that come with being physically fit. On the other hand, if your workout regimen consists of twelve-ounce curls and occasional brisk walks to the trash dumpster and back, it's time for you to get motivated.

When it comes to working out, it's nice to have a partner. So if your woman is already exercising regularly, why not join her? Or if she's not already with the program, try persuading her to get involved. The benefits of exercise for an expectant mom can be huge during pregnancy, delivery, and postpartum recovery.

If your woman already leads an active lifestyle of which regular exercise is a component, being pregnant shouldn't keep her from continuing her exercise routine, although the more hard-core female athlete may need to tone down her activities when she is with child. That can mean no contact sports or extreme sports, at least until she gets clearance from her doctor following childbirth.

If she hasn't exercised regularly prior to conception, pregnancy may be a good time for her to start. In fact, fitness experts and groups such as the American College of Obstetricians and Gynecologists recommend that pregnant women exercise several times a week, not to lose weight but to be more fit for the next three trimesters and beyond.

Following a regular exercise routine that includes cardiovascular activity, strength training, and/or stretching provides perks to both of you. Benefits for the pregnant woman include:

- Increased flexibility, balance, and resiliency

- Help staying within the targeted range for weight gain during pregnancy (she should ask her doctor what her target range is)

- Increased energy level and stamina

- Strengthened bones and muscles so they are better equipped to endure the added burden of childbearing

- Lessened impact of such pregnancy-related conditions as constipation, muscle cramping, and swelling

- Improved circulation

- An outlet for reducing stress and fatigue

- Relaxation, perhaps leading to better sleep

With so much on his plate during pregnancy, the sedentary caveman may be ambivalent about starting a workout regimen. He may be a bit wary about working out alongside his woman for fear she will force him into compromising yoga or pilates poses and embarrassing aerobic dance classes that expose his rhythmic shortcomings. He may fear that even in her third trimester, she'll still complete the three-mile jogging loop before he does. While competition can be healthy in driving one another to a higher level of fitness, your chief goal isn't to win any races but rather just to get (or stay) in shape. With that in mind, it's healthy to develop a routine in which the two of you exercise separately as well as together.

"Not so fast," the unmotivated skeptic in you says. "I haven't agreed to be part of this."

Here it's worth pointing out that the caveman also stands to reap significant benefits by supplementing couch time and parental preparations with regular exercise. Like his woman, he will have activities that increase strength, endurance, flexibility, and overall health. He'll feel better about himself and his physique. And he and his woman will establish that sweaty kind of bond only shared by workout partners. So rather than taking the easy route to weight loss—liposuction, gastric bypass (a.k.a. stomach-stapling)—why not take the higher, harder road to a less lumpy figure?

EXERCISE CAUTION

Before embarking on an exercise program, it's advisable for your woman to ask her doctor to provide some safe parameters for prenatal workouts. A personal trainer or fitness expert who is experienced in designing workout programs for pregnant women also can help set those parameters. They may suggest she reduce the intensity of workouts late in pregnancy.

When it comes to partners exercising together, keep in mind that the pregnant half of the partnership will need to monitor her body's behavior during physical activity much more closely than the caveman will need to monitor his. There are limits to what a pregnant woman should subject herself to while exercising. For example, she should avoid exercises that jar, rattle, or bounce her body or put her at risk of falling—activities such as downhill skiing, horseback riding, waterskiing, snowboarding, surfing, rugby, rock climbing, and skydiving.

AIN'T NO STOPPING US NOW

Absent any medical conditions that may preclude a woman from exercising during pregnancy (and there are several, as Dr. Brian points out on p. 111), there's nothing to keep her from working out and stretching at least every other day—and as often as every day—as long as the activity isn't too strenuous or dangerous. For the vast majority of pregnant women, it's fine to:

- **SWIM**
- **WALK**
- **JOG**
- **HIKE**
- **BIKE**
- **AEROBICIZE**
- **PLAY TENNIS**
- **USE A CARDIO MACHINE** such as a stair-stepper, stationary bike or elliptical
- **PLAY GOLF**

- **LIFT WEIGHTS** (two to three times per week maximum)
- **DO YOGA OR PILATES** (not all kinds are suited to a woman with child)
- **CROSS-COUNTRY SKI**

EQUIPMENT

For months you have been hemorrhaging money on baby gear. Now a newfound zest for physical activity affords the expectant couple the opportunity to spend some cash on themselves for a change. Here are some of the items on Gronk's workout wish list: heart monitor; running/walking shoes; hiking shoes/boots; sports bra (woman only, unless her partner has developed man-boobs as part of his sympathetic pregnancy); athletic supporter (to keep the cavejewels in place); breathable, nonrestrictive clothes; foul-weather wear; a hat to shade your head; sunscreen; the means to hydrate (water bottle, hydration pack); a yoga or exercise mat (for stretching, yoga, etc.); light dumbbell weights; a pack to store snacks for an activity of longer duration; a diary or calendar to track you and your partner's progress (weight loss/gain, workout duration, etc.); a health-club membership (if you prefer not working out at home); a workout/yoga/pilates video or DVD; an iPod or other type of personal music device and earphones that stay in your ears when you start sweating; other activity-specific equipment—swim goggles, cross-country skis, a bicycle (with a comfy saddle designed specially for the female anatomy), golf clubs, tennis racket, etc.

MAKE JANE FONDA AND RICHARD SIMMONS PROUD

The doctor has cleared your partner to start an exercise program. You have summoned the mental resolve to join her in the program. The gear has been purchased. The will is there. Now it's time to start exercising in earnest. This needn't be viewed as a huge commitment: even thirty minutes a day of sustained physical activity, three times a week, will yield positive results, especially for those who up to this point haven't been exercising at all.

That sounds enticing. But how to begin? A prenatal exercise regimen consists of three basic components: stretching, cardiovascular exercise, and strength training.

STRETCHING Your arms are disproportionately long, but you still can't get your hairy knuckles to touch your toes because your hamstrings are as tight as guitar strings. To the caveman, that's a sign it's time to begin a stretching program as part of an overall workout regimen.

But don't forget, this is more about your woman than you. A regular stretching routine not only will help your flexibility, it can do wonders for a pregnant woman as well. Stretching, like exercise, reduces muscle tension, boosts circulation, enhances relaxation, and helps avoid injury. And for expectant mothers, it can help prepare the muscles around the midsection and pelvis for the trauma of childbirth while also lessening pregnancy-related discomfort in areas such as the joints and the back. A

doctor and/or trainer can provide ideas for stretches and exercises designed specifically for moms-to-be—pelvic tilts, wall stretches, wall squats, back flexions, among others.

One thing to keep in mind: during pregnancy, the body releases a hormone called relaxin that loosens ligaments. While that's generally a good thing because it provides more flexibility to let the baby come through the birth canal, the presence of more relaxin also can make joints more susceptible to injury. To combat that, women with child should:

▸ Emphasize stretches that incorporate slow, easy movements

▸ Avoid those that require sharp, jerky, or high-impact movements

▸ Avoid pushing a stretch to the point where it becomes painful

▸ Stretch after a brief warm-up, not when the muscles are cold

▸ Stretch after concluding a workout

CARDIOVASCULAR EXERCISE These are activities that strengthen the body's cardiovascular system—heart, lungs, arteries, veins, and capillaries. What's great about "cardio" exercise is that it can give the two of you a good workout in a relatively short period of time, through a wide range of beneficial activities, from cross-country skiing to swimming. A workout regimen that includes cardio as a major component will boost endurance and circulation, reduce the incidence of varicose veins appearing after childbirth (a somewhat common and potentially unsightly side effect of the birthing process), and generally improve a person's sense of physical well being.

If neither of you is accustomed to regular exercise, no need to be heroes to begin with. Start slow and build up to higher intensity cardio workouts (without overdoing it, of course—monitor your lady's heart rate).

STRENGTH TRAINING While weightlifting isn't especially prevalent among pregnant women, it's perfectly safe during pregnancy as long as the woman takes special precautions and exercises restraint. That's where her workout partner can play an important role.

Your woman doesn't want her sweaty, tank-top-clad partner hovering over her on the bench press, exhorting her to "max out." Just the opposite. A low-weight, low-impact program is the smartest strength-training strategy for expectant moms.

Still, there may be better methods than pumping iron for a pregnant woman to achieve her fitness goals. So before she shoehorns her expanding body into a spandex outfit and heads to the buffeteria, she should consult with her doctor, then perhaps with a personal trainer or fitness expert who has a strong background in prenatal strength training.

Whether heading out for a light jog or to the golf course to play nine holes, pregnant women (and their workout partners) should take precautions to protect themselves and their babies from problems. That means:

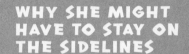

DR. BRIAN

WHY SHE MIGHT HAVE TO STAY ON THE SIDELINES

Beyond his typical motor-skill and muscular-coordination challenges, there is little to hold back the healthy caveman sweathog in his workout activities. That's not the case with some expectant moms, however. Certain health conditions can force a pregnant woman to avoid exercise because it may increase the risk of preterm labor and/or endanger her health and that of the fetus, among them:

▶ **HIGH BLOOD PRESSURE**

▶ **PREECLAMPSIA**

▶ **HEART PROBLEMS**

▶ **DIABETES**

▶ **HISTORY OF SEIZURES**

▶ **PHENYLKETONURIA (PKU)**

▶ **EATING DISORDERS**

DR. BRIAN

THE UNSUNG EXERCISE: TONING THE PUBOCOCCYGEUS

The medical community sees them merely as a means to keep the muscles at the base of the pelvis, around the vagina, anus, and urethra in good working condition. But there is more to Kegel exercises than that. For women, "Kegels" are a way to keep a certain key muscle toned. For the caveman, they are a source of mystery and wonder. His simple mind is intrigued by the idea that such an important muscle can be exercised without any outward sign of activity. It's eye-opening when he discovers exactly what Kegel exercises are and the potential far-reaching benefits they provide to regular practitioners—both female and male. The exercises, named after the late American gynecologist (and contemporary caveman role model) Arnold H. Kegel, are meant to increase the strength and resilience of the pubococcygeus muscle. You have one down there in the pubic region and so does your woman. And having a toned one can benefit both of you. For example, a woman who regularly does Kegel exercises may enjoy:

- An easier labor

- A quicker recovery from an episiotomy

- Less discomfort during pelvic exams

- And perhaps of special interest to you: greater pleasure during intercourse, since it is believed in medical circles that strengthening the "PC" muscle increases the chances of women achieving orgasm

In fact, you may want to join in her Kegel exercise regimen. It is also believed that men who do the exercises regularly may be able to sustain erections longer. So for a few minutes each day performing Kegel moves called "flicks" and "elevators," you can accomplish naturally what would otherwise require a little pill.

- Hydrating by drinking plenty of water before, during, and after exercise

- Having a snack before exercising to provide your body with fuel for the workout

- Trying not to overheat. Avoid working out in hot or humid weather and wear breathable clothing that keeps you cool. In bright sunshine, wear a hat.

- Being aware that her balance may be upset because her center of gravity has shifted with a baby onboard

- Not pushing a workout too far. Doctors advise pregnant women to keep their heart rate in check, so have her use a heart monitor or her own finger to check her pulse while exercising. If her heart rate exceeds the maximum level recommended by her doctor (typically 140 beats per minute), she should take a break, and when/if she resumes activity, she should dial down the intensity a notch or two.

- Watching for signs of trouble. Conditions such as dizziness/lightheadedness, shortness of breath, irregular heartbeat, vaginal bleeding, and uterine contractions that arise during or after exercise are red flags indicating it's time to stop the workout and call the doctor.

CHAPTER 6

CAVEMAN COOKS FOR THREE (OR MORE)

*Above all, do not fail to give good dinners,
and to pay attention to the women.*

—NAPOLEAN BONAPARTE

THE QUESTION HAS crossed your primitive mind more than once: why aren't we all Neanderthals? Here's why:

Some 30,000 years ago the species known as Neanderthal man (*Homo neanderthalensis*) mysteriously died out while its cavedwelling counterpart, the Cro-Magnon, one of our early *Homo sapiens* ancestors, somehow managed to persevere through

GROW WITH GRONK

What the caveman stands to gain from reading Chapter 6:

➧ **POWER** to positively influence the health and nutrition of his woman and baby

➧ **A LIFELONG SKILL** to set him apart from his prehistoric peers

➧ **GREAT APPRECIATION** from all who dine on his meals

➧ **A WORKING KNOWLEDGE** of the Do-No-Harm principles of caveman cooking

➧ **A FIRM KNOWLEDGE** of the nutrients woman and fetus need for good health and growth

➧ **THE KNOW-HOW** to navigate modern hunting and gathering grounds in search of ingredients

➧ **STRATEGIES** for catering to a pregnant woman's food cravings and aversions

➧ **THE ABILITY** to follow safe food handling practices and prepare meals without poisoning anyone

➧ **THE SMARTS** to convert teaspoons to tablespoons, ounces to grams

➧ **THE SKILLS** to grill, roast, bake, boil, brew, toss, marinate, mix, and otherwise prepare awe-inspiring meals and drinks

the endless winter of the Pleistocene period. Even today, the debate rages among prehistorians and evolutionary scholars as to why Cro-Magnon man survived but Neanderthal man didn't. Some claim it was dietary shortcomings that wreaked havoc on the Neanderthal species. The oversized brow and other physical features common to Neanderthals, they posit, could be the manifestation of an iodine deficiency akin to a condition we now call cretinism. Ultimately, that dietary deficiency may have led to extinction.

The brutishly browed Neanderthals, who roamed parts of Europe and Asia for roughly 200,000 years, were known to be skilled big-game hunters and voracious meat eaters. So why didn't those traits translate into longevity? Perhaps the key to Cro-Magnons outlasting their prehistoric compadres was their diverse diet. Cro-Magnons were proficient hunters and gatherers, omnivores who ate plants in addition to fish and game. The fossil record indicates that later generations of Cro-Magnons not only knew how to slay large and small game, drag it back to the cave, butcher the carcass, and cook it over a firepit, they could also forage for nuts, berries, and whatever other herbaceous delicacies they found on the desolate tundra. They could make square meals that provided them with the sustenance and nutritional content necessary to endure under adverse environmental conditions, while their Neanderthal cousins fell by the evolutionary wayside.

Here in the twenty-first century, an expectant father who lacks the complete kitchen package—hunting, gathering, and cooking skills—could face a fate similar to that of the Neanderthal. When it comes to kitchen proficiency, many members of the male species might be mistaken for well-embrowed Neanderthals. While these guys may be skilled big-game hunters, savvy open-flame cooks, and highly accomplished carnivores, they can't gather and prepare all the ingredients for a nutritiously balanced meal to save their lives. Left to their own devices, these contemporary cavemen would gladly subsist on a diet of prepared, delivered, or scavenged food.

With a baby on the way, the lives of your woman and unborn child now depend on you evolving beyond one-dimensional Neanderthal ways. To be a viable partner in the pregnancy venture, you need to bring diverse culinary skills to the table. For the expectant mother and womb-bound baby, a steady diet of ramen noodles, frozen pizzas, and Chinese take-out simply will not do. The situation demands that the expectant father emerge from his culinary cave, don an apron, and assume his rightful place in the kitchen. This isn't a bad thing. In fact, it's a great opportunity to evolve into a cultivated caveman chef, one who can turn what he hunts and gathers into excellent meals fit for the changing dietary requirements and tastes of his pregnant mate. So rather than balk at the idea, why not embrace it? You have much to gain and little to lose by learning to hold your own in the kitchen. Best of all, you'll be acquiring a lifelong skill that you can not only use yourself but pass on to your kids, even your grandchildren. Now is the time to seize the opportunity, since you'll be short on time and energy once the baby arrives. With a prehistoric partner to cook with her and for her, your mate will have more time for activities, exercise, and relaxation, three crucial ingredients for a healthy, less stressful pregnancy. For you, it's a ticket to self-sufficiency in the kitchen. Take the stuff in this chapter seriously and you'll be able to deliver tasty meals cooked especially to meet the distinct nutritional needs—and ever-shifting tastes—of a pregnant woman. But the benefits that come with your newfound culinary prowess aren't limited to the pregnancy period, nor to just the female sex. The meals you make will taste so good you'll want to keep cooking once your child arrives. And it will be important for you to keep cooking, as the days of frequent dining out are coming to an end. Becoming proficient in the kitchen is also a genuine opportunity to become a positive force in the health of your family. You spend much of pregnancy in a supporting role. But here you can seize the rare opportunity to actively and positively influence the health of two humans other than yourself.

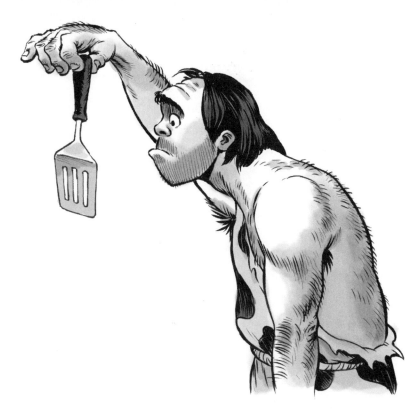

Roughly four million women give birth each year in the United States. Not a single one of them would complain if the men in their lives were to share cooking duties during pregnancy. So many pregnant women and so many pregnancy-related books, yet mysteriously, so little is written to specifically empower expectant fathers with kitchen skills so they can relieve their mates of sole meal-making responsibilities.

If men were the ones who bore children, you can bet that the shelves would be crammed with books written specifically to make their lives easier during pregnancy. Yet here in the real world, where women do the childbearing, most books written for expectant parents do surprisingly little to relieve women of their kitchen responsibilities at a time when they need relief most. This chapter introduces the expectant father to essential gathering tips, cooking techniques, kitchen strategies, and recipes. They will help you on your path to culinary proficiency, while providing your woman with a steady diet of healthy, nutritious meals and snacks designed especially for her prenatal needs and palate. This journey, if embraced with gusto, is sure to enrich and reward the caveman and all who dine at his table.

PONDER THIS

COOKING WITH ALCOHOL

What happens when the caveman is cooking for a pregnant woman and the recipe calls for alcohol (such as wine or brandy)? Whether you follow the recipe and include the alcohol depends on (a) if the woman is abstaining altogether from alcohol consumption during pregnancy; (b) how much alcohol the recipe calls for; and (c) the extent to which the alcohol will be allowed to "cook off." If she prefers not to let alcohol touch her lips, leave it out of the recipe (which could make the end result less palatable) or find another nonalcoholic recipe to cook. If she's open to eating foods containing a small amount of alcohol, work from recipes that call for simmering, a cooking technique that allows most but not all the alcohol to cook off.

THE HIPPOCRATIC OATH FOR CAVECOOKS

Let food be thy medicine and medicine be thy food.

—HIPPOCRATES

Hippocrates, a cultivated caveman from way back in the fifth century BC, was right on the mark when he made the connection between food and medicine. Hailed as the father of medicine, he lived to the ripe old age of eighty-three, a testament perhaps to his healthy eating habits.

The Hippocratic Oath, drafted around 400 BC, was named after the Grecian Hippocrates because by historical accounts he either wrote the oath himself or helped shape its contents. Today the oath is as relevant as ever, serving as the ethical code for modern medicine. One of the main tenets espoused by the toga-clad father of medicine (though not explicitly in the Hippocratic Oath) was the principle "Do no harm."

"As to diseases," Hippocrates wrote in his treatise *Epidemics*, "make a habit of two things—to help, or at least to do no harm."

Think you're not cut out to be a cook? Follow the three Do-No-Harm principles of caveman cooking listed below, learn a few basic cooking techniques, use fresh ingredients, and you will be well on your way to transforming yourself into a meal-making maestro.

PRINCIPLE 1:
DO NO HARM TO THOSE YOU SERVE

Always follow safe food-handling practices—cooking meats to the proper temperature, cooking ground meats thoroughly, avoiding cross-contamination (such as from handling raw meat then slicing a loaf a bread without washing your hands in between), and washing produce (fruits, vegetables, etc.) thoroughly.

PRINCIPLE 2:
DO NO HARM TO THYSELF

You're doing no one any favors, particularly not your pregnant woman, if you get hauled away to the hospital in a meat wagon because you nearly severed a digit while haphazardly handling a knife. So protect your extremities when using sharp kitchen instruments. Cut especially long locks, use a hairnet, or else exercise extra care to see that those locks don't get tangled in kitchen appliances such as the mixer or get burned by the stovetop flame. Also remember to wear an oven mitt, lest you singe the hair on your palms. And don't burn down the building; pay attention to what you're cooking, especially with meals involving an open flame or hot oil. Fire is a relatively new concept to you, so it's wise to keep a fire extinguisher close just in case. Also, you may want to avoid flambé recipes until your kitchen skills and handling of fire are more polished.

PRINCIPLE 3:
DO NO HARM TO YOUR RELATIONSHIP

What good is a caveman cook if he's leaving his woman with a mountain of dishes to wash after preparing a meal? When you're working in the kitchen, wash, rinse, and put away dishes and instruments as you go. This approach gives you more room to maneuver—a major consideration when cooking in a cramped space—and relieves your woman and you of postmeal dish duty.

STOCKING THE PRENATAL PANTRY: HEALTHY HUNTING & GATHERING HABITS

We are living in a world today where lemonade is made from artificial flavors and furniture polish is made from real lemons.

—ALFRED E. NEWMAN

Your hunting, gathering, and gastronomic routine is among many facets of life that will change now that you're expecting. Your pregnant lady (and the baby growing inside her) has very specific nutritional needs, and her tastes likely will change frequently and without warning as she advances through pregnancy. Foods that tasted good to her in the first trimester may turn her stomach in the second or third. (Word of warning: don't be surprised if she sends you to the couch for the night if her keen pregnant-lady nose detects one of those offending foods on your breath).

As her new culinary cohort, you are now entrusted with cooking meals that not only appeal to her ever-changing palate, but also meet her dietary requirements. Not to worry. All the recipes included here were designed with those needs in mind. What's more, they have been carefully vetted by Kelli, a member of the Expectant Caveman's Ad Hoc Female Advisory Council, and more importantly, a registered dietician with specialized training in the prenatal nutritional needs of women. Her dietary and nutritional wisdom is sprinkled like a fine imported spice throughout this chapter.

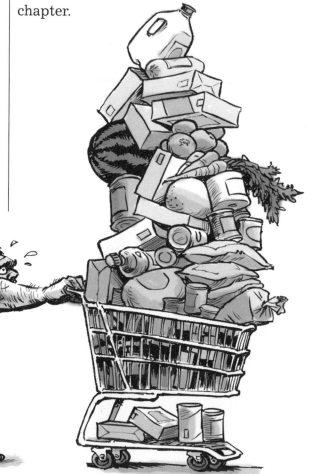

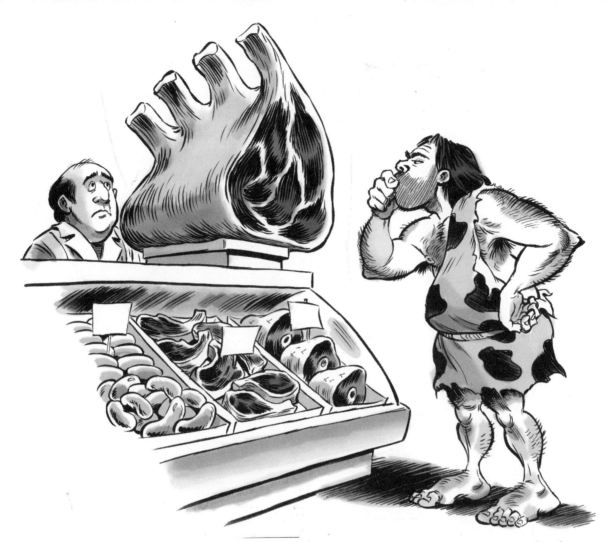

As the expectant mom advances through pregnancy, her dietary needs will change along with her tastes. She is going to need to consume at least three hundred to four hundred more calories a day throughout pregnancy to keep herself going and the baby growing. This added energy shouldn't come from a couple of chicken nuggets with ranch dressing, but rather from a well-balanced diet containing a wide variety of foods that offer nutritional value, not just junk calories.

Our Cro-Magnon ancestors would be astounded by the grocery stores of today—the produce watering system, droning muzak, broad aisles stacked high with cans and boxes, and so many different scents to overwhelm the senses. Even today, guys with slightly protruding brows who are accustomed to foraging for food at convenience stores can find themselves confused in these environs. But because taking on meal-making responsibilities entails also hunting and gathering to stock your home and kitchen with ingredients for your culinary creations, you now must frequent such places as grocery stores, specialty food stores, weekend farmers' markets, and roadside produce stands. Effectively navigating these places means making out a list of what to buy ahead of time, knowing where to find the items on that list, and asking uniformed store personnel when an item cannot be located. Cavemen who are skilled enough to grow their own crops have another fresh source of ingredients that won't require a perilous journey to the grocery store.

When loping through the aisles of this new hunting ground, the caveman's mind drifts to thoughts of his Cro-Magnon ancestors. He pictures them hungrily searching for fresh fruits and vegetables, climbing, digging, and risking life and limb to find the best and ripest of the bunch. When the Cro-Magnon finds something to

his liking, he hoists his prize toward the sky, chanting and screaming in homage to the goddess of fertility while warding off rival cavemen who covet the same bounty.

That kind of display won't be tolerated in the grocery store produce aisle, you are told by the in-store rent-a-cop as he rips the bananas from your clutches. Having regained your composure, you glance down the aisle at a wide woman in a floral-pattern muumuu, reading the nutritional contents on a bag of baked potato chips. Later you notice the gossip magazines at the checkout

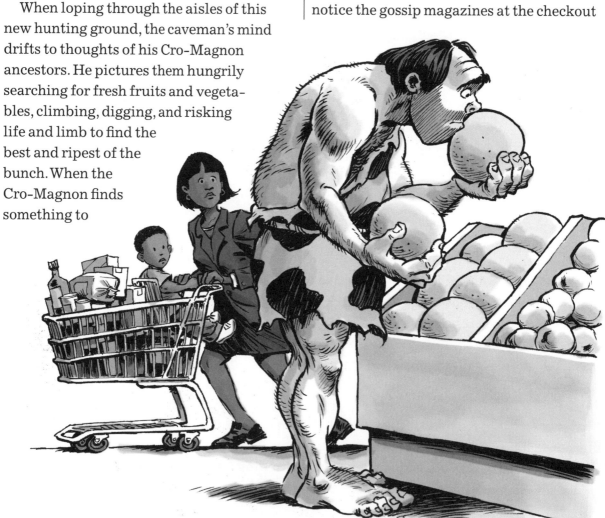

COOKIN' FOR THE PREGNANT BELLY WITH KELLI

ANTIDOTES TO MORNING MISERY

About three in four pregnant women will battle nausea—morning sickness—at some point during their term. There is no known cause for morning sickness, nor is there a surefire way to cure it. But there are effective ways for the caveman cook to help treat the condition, which usually affects women during the first trimester. The spice ginger (not to be confused with Ginger Spice of the Spice Girls, who has been known to cause nausea, not cure it) has been shown to be an effective ingredient in battling the queasy belly without the use of drugs. So a food as innocuous as store-bought ginger snaps may be just what your woman needs to chase away the greenness. You can buy fresh ginger (as a root) in the produce aisle of your local grocery store or specialty food shop, then use it to make a sheet of gingerbread, put in a smoothie, or use in an Asian stir-fry.

To ease her morning (or more likely, all-day) sickness, also try:

➤ The Rise and Dine approach, in which you leave a plate of crackers on her bedside table at night so she can snack on a couple when she wakes in the morning. This gives her an immediate means of restoring some of the nutrients her body passed to the fetus while she slept.

➤ Keeping strong odors (from food and other sources, so yes, do use deodorant) to a minimum

➤ Avoiding greasy, fried, and overseasoned foods

➤ Providing her with cold, nonsmelly foods such as smoothies, crackers, plain bread, and cold cereal

➤ Keeping freshly cut lemon slices handy; their scent can calm the tummy

➤ Suggesting she take her prenatal vitamin at night if taking it at other times of the day causes nausea. This may allow her to sleep through most of the discomfort.

COOKIN' FOR THE PREGNANT BELLY WITH KELL

BACK OFF BOILING AND SKINNING

Overcooked, skinned veggies can't match their crunchy counterparts in nutritional value. Boiling veggies can actually allow their water-soluble vitamins (vitamins B and C) to escape into the water. Also, when you remove skins and seeds, you are removing valuable fiber and wasting valuable time. So give items like carrots, potatoes, and cucumbers a good scrubbin' but leave on their skins. Rule of thumb: fresh and fibrous is best, but if you don't want them raw, try steaming or sautéing.

counter are full of stories—all absolutely true—about the travails of overweight and unhealthy celebrities. What the tabloid gossip rags won't tell you is that obesity and diabetes are at record levels in the United States. Why is that the case, when dieting and diet foods abound at grocery stores? Why does it seem as if people are eschewing the products nature provides in favor of over-hyped, undernourishing faddish foods?

The unfortunate answer is that so-called fast food and processed foods have become staples of the modern diet. People have forgotten or ignored the fact that the further removed food is from its natural state, the more additives it contains and the less healthy it is to ingest.

Living off the land, ranging far and wide in harsh conditions over unforgiving terrain in search of the ingredients in their diet, our cavedwelling forebears were often confronted with the problem of finding enough food for everyone in the clan. That's a far cry from the cavemen of today, who are more apt to grapple with *too many* food options, not enough of which are healthy to eat. Sure, the Cro-Magnon could die from a common cold, but at least the corpse he left behind was fit, trim, and once decomposed, a good source of nutrients for the soil.

When foraging in the hunting and gathering grounds of today, the caveman should leave room in his wheeled chariot for plenty of foods that are still in their natural, unprocessed state. Gather fruits, vegetables, and nuts and leave the prepackaged snack cakes in aisle 47, where they have sat moldering since the last millennium. These natural foods are good to have around the house as meal ingredients and as stand-alone snacks. Shopping the perimeter of the grocery store gives you the best chance to find foods in their most natural and healthiest state. Even though you may occasionally need to dart into an aisle for an item, you will find most of your natural, unprocessed, healthy foods on the perimeter.

The benefits of healthy eating and home cooking extend past the soon-to-be-mom and soon-to-be-infant you are intending to help. See the guy in the mirror with a huge stress load and expanding belt line? With so many projects to take care of, maybe he hasn't been taking care of himself by getting out to exercise as much as he should. Perhaps he's having an extra "coping" beer or two at night while eating too much of the food from aisle 47. That's right, Mr. Primitive Palate, cutting out the junk food not only helps mom and baby, but it can also keep you from packing on the sympathy pounds and achieving artery-popping cholesterol levels.

As a new father, you can count on having less time, energy, and disposable income to eat out frequently. So making home-cooked meals also benefits a budget that may otherwise be depleted by baby-related activities and gear. The money you save in eating out less can go right to the newborn's day care needs or college fund. Rather than lamenting your less frequent restaurant visits, why not revel in your newfound domesticity by making an effort to enjoy the additional time you are spending in the kitchen and at home with your new addition?

FOOD FOR THE FICKLE PALATE: CATERING TO A PREGNANT WOMAN'S CRAVINGS

As an accomplished late-night-television channel surfer, you surely have seen pregnant female characters in those outdated family sitcoms subsisting on mass quantities of pickles and ice cream. In some cases this

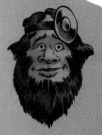

DR. BRIAN

PICA-BOO

You hope what you just witnessed was a hallucination. What you thought you saw defies logic: your woman stops in her tracks, glances this way and that, then furtively dips her hand into a ceramic planter, grabs a heaping helping of potting soil, shovels it into her mouth, chews, and swallows. Has she just enthusiastically consumed a fistful of enriched dirt? If so, her motive for wolfing it down may not have been to purge her mouth of the lingering taste of your chicken kebabs, but rather the manifestation of an extremely rare, potentially dangerous medical condition known as pica (pronounced pie-kuh). Medically, pica (Latin for magpie, a bird that will eat almost anything) is described as a disorder that drives a pregnant woman to crave non-food—and often unhealthy and even life-threatening—substances, from household goods like laundry detergent to plain old dirt. It is not known for certain why some women develop pica cravings during pregnancy. There is currently no identified cause; however, according to the Journal of American Dietetic Association there may be a connection to iron deficiency. Pica cravings are most commonly seen in children and occur in approximately 1.5 percent of all children. Pica-type cravings of pregnant women are even less common, but not abnormal. These cravings gone wild make baking soda, clay, and other odd items seem like a pretty exciting multicourse meal. If you spot signs that your woman has these strange urges ("Why is she gnawing on my flip-flop?"), don't panic. Call a health care provider, monitor the vitamin and mineral intake of your partner, and consider suggesting potential substitutes for her cravings such as sugarless chewing gum.

PONDER THIS

LET IT FLOW

Water covers two-thirds of the earth and constitutes about two-thirds of the typical person's bodyweight, so it is no wonder women should consume plenty of it during pregnancy. In fact, a pregnant woman's water intake should increase right along with her caloric intake. Fluids help the body absorb nutrients and produce some of the building blocks of life: new cells and blood. So, caveman, be sure your pregnant woman drinks enough fluids—and enough water in particular.

stereotype is grounded in reality, as pregnant women are known to have acute and sometimes bizarre cravings, especially in the first trimester.

Ask any caveman who's lived with a pregnant woman and he will tell you that her tastes for given foods, flavors, and ingredients can be fickle. Foods she craved prior to pregnancy she may not tolerate now. Certain especially pungent ingredients, such as onions and garlic, may provoke a strong negative reaction, while certain other ingredients can spark an equally strong attraction. Further, those aversions and attractions are constantly moving targets. Something she likes one month may turn her stomach the next.

As a caveman cook trying to cater to a pregnant woman's needs, don't burn too many brain cells trying to make sense of her

cravings; you're best off accepting them and moving forward with whatever meal you're making, minus any ingredients she finds offensive at this point during pregnancy.

Some people posit that the food cravings women experience while pregnant are the body's and the baby's way of saying they need foods with specific nutrients. While this theory has never been proven, it sounds logical to the caveman's simplistic way of thinking. Science tells us that cravings actually are a by-product of hormonal changes and with many women, they will dissipate sometime around the fourth month of pregnancy.

If your woman is eating a diet containing the vitamins and ingredients that are crucial to prenatal nutrition (we'll go into those in a moment), the occasional indulgence with foods commonly found in the donut aisle of the supermarket can't really hurt. Indeed, such a junk-food foray may be valuable merely for the immediate gratification it provides. But for the most part, as a pregnant woman's caveman caterer, your job is to stock the fridge and cupboards with foods that provide the ingredients your mate needs to be at her healthiest.

In the rarest cases, a woman's cravings may veer toward extremely strange and potentially unhealthy desires for nonfood items found around the home and yard. If you notice boxes of laundry soap piling up in the garbage and the occasional bubble wafting out of your woman's mouth as she speaks, she may have a real and serious disorder called pica (see Dr. Brian: Pica-Boo, p. 123).

Our first instinct in writing this book was to steer our recipes toward the carnivore. But common sense and input from the enlightened members of our Female Advisory Council dictated that we not neglect the significant segment of the populace representing herbivores—vegetarians. Most herbivores that prehistoric man encountered walked on four or more legs and ate leaves from the tops of thirty-foot shrubs. So it is understandably difficult at times for the modern caveman of today, who has carried on the meat-eating tradition of his ancestors, to fathom a meatless (sometimes even a dairyless) diet. But if your woman is a vegetarian or vegan, you need to prepare meals accordingly rather than attempt to force your carnivorous ways upon her.

BUILDING BLOCKS FOR A HEALTHY PRENATAL DIET

Variety is the spice of life. And in the case of a woman's prenatal diet, variety will almost always provide the proper mix of nutrients that she and the baby require.

Why make the effort to cook nutritiously? Because a healthy mom often translates into a healthy baby. For growth, the fetus depends on nutrients the pregnant woman supplies, so a nutritious prenatal diet for the expectant mother means a good gestational diet for the baby. Eating well also gives a

COOKIN' FOR THE PREGNANT BELLY WITH KELLI

ONE-TWO PUNCH

Although a pregnant woman absorbs iron at three times her normal nonpregnant rate, her body still needs help. Vitamin C encourages the body to absorb iron, so it's a good idea to serve her foods and drinks containing vitamin C as an accompaniment to iron-rich foods. For example, serve orange juice with whole-grain cereal, add lime juice to cooked ground meat, and add bell peppers to whole-grain pasta. Other foods rich in vitamin C include strawberries, cantaloupe, grapefruit, and broccoli.

woman much-needed energy during pregnancy while lessening the chance she'll go into premature labor. And once she has the baby, a good diet will better equip her body to bounce back from birth.

Here are a few of the vitamins, minerals, and nutrients most important to fetal development:

IRON. Because of changes in your woman's body during pregnancy, she needs twice the amount of iron that she did prior to pregnancy. When a woman is with child, her blood volume increases 25 percent. Iron is

COOKIN' FOR THE PREGNANT BELLY WITH KELLI

WHOLE GRAIN GOOD

When hunting for carb sources, look for ones with the highest fiber content. Focus on using grain products that are composed of 100 percent whole grain.

Your woman has a higher risk of encountering the dreaded condition called constipation and needs extra fiber and water to stay happy, healthy, and habitual.

essential to development of hemoglobin, which carries oxygen in the blood to both woman and fetus. It also helps combat infection and fatigue. Since it is nearly impossible for a pregnant woman to meet her daily iron requirement from meals alone, an iron supplement is usually prescribed (see "Cookin' for the Pregnant Belly With Kelli" on p. 128 for more information on dietary supplements). Sources include lean red meat, spinach, tofu, dried fruit, whole-grain breads, and cereals (not the kind with marshmallows in them).

CALCIUM. A woman's calcium requirement also doubles during pregnancy, to about 1,200 milligrams per day. The *in utero* caveling needs that calcium throughout pregnancy for the formation of strong bones and teeth. Gnawing on bones discarded by the local butcher shop won't do the trick. For calcium sources that are easier on the teeth, your woman can turn to foods such as dairy products (milk, cheese, yogurt), dried beans, collard greens, and broccoli. If your woman doesn't do dairy, it is important that you find her other good sources of calcium. Some alternatives include calcium-fortified orange juice, fortified soymilk, fortified soy yogurt, fortified rice milk, and tofu processed with calcium sulfate.

PROTEIN. A prenatal diet should offer plenty of protein, the main building block for fetal cells. Doctors generally recommend that women elevate their protein intake to about sixty grams per day. Not only does protein promote growth of fetal cells, but it also bolsters blood supply and provides energy reserves to both the woman and the baby. Eggs, lean meats, fish, cheese, milk, and beans are excellent sources of protein. For the woman who prefers a nonmeat diet or craves something spongy, tofu is also a good source of protein. Generally speaking, the firmer the tofu, the more protein and calcium it contains (check amounts of calcium sulfate on the package to see exactly how much calcium is in there). Made from boiled bean curd, tofu can be added to cold dishes and to drinks such as smoothies, or it can be the featured protein in a full-blown hot meal.

MEATER READER

Protein good. Math bad. Here's a cheat sheet for the numerically challenged caveman to calculate protein per servings of common foods.

FOOD SOURCE	SERVING SIZE	PROTEIN PER SERVING
Meat/poultry/fish	3 oz cooked	21 g
Eggs	1 lg	7 g
Milk	8 oz	8 g
Yogurt (plain)	1 cup	9 g
Tofu (firm)	4 oz	8 g
Peanut butter	1 tbsp	4 g
Cottage cheese	2/3 cup	20 g
Beans (lentils, black, chick peas, etc.)	1½ cups	20 g
Cheese (Swiss, cheddar, etc.)	3 oz	20 g

CARBOHYDRATES. While some of today's fad diets steer people away from carbs, pregnant women should be steering toward them. Carbohydrates provide energy to woman and fetus alike, while helping protein perform one of its key tasks during pregnancy: promoting fetal tissue growth. Sources of good carbs include whole-grain and fortified breads and cereals, fruits, vegetables, rice, pasta, and potatoes.

FATS. Fad diets also tend to characterize all fats as unhealthy. That's not the case, though. Healthy forms of fat provide the fetus with energy reserves for growth and are critical to development of the fetal brain, skin, and vision. While fats make up an important component of a healthy diet, all fats are not created equal, and therefore, it's up to you, the caveman cook, to keep an eye on the fat content of the foods you prepare. Certain fats, such as monounsaturated and polyunsaturated, have a favorable effect on blood cholesterol levels. They are primarily found in liquid form in vegetable oils, such as olive oil. On the other hand, saturated fats, such as those found in shortening (and french fries, see "Ponder This" on p. 159), usually come in solid form at room temperature and should be consumed in moderation. Also limit her intake of transfatty acids (trans fats), which can negatively impact blood cholesterol levels. In general, any processed food is a potential source of trans fats. But take heart, because when you fill your grocery store chariot with foods in their natural state, you are steering clear of harmful amounts of transfatty acids. In addition to olive oil, good sources of monounsaturated and polyunsaturated fats include lean meat, fish, poultry, eggs, nuts, seeds, and peanut butter. Yogurt and mozzarella cheese sticks are snacks that offer healthier forms of fat.

FOLIC ACID. Folic acid fosters red blood cell and hemoglobin formation while also helping prevent neural tube defects in the fetus. Sources include dark, leafy greens such as spinach, citrus fruits, bananas, tomatoes, and whole-grain breads and cereals.

COOKIN' FOR THE PREGNANT BELLY WITH KELLI

PRENATAL VITAMINS

Flintstones brand multivitamins are great for cavemen but what about for their pregnant women? If one vitamin is good, more is better, right? Wrong! Although it is important that your woman take a prenatal vitamin, doubling up or routinely adding extra vitamins to the diet can be harmful. For example, vitamin A is crucial to fetal development, but ingesting too much of it from supplements, fortified foods, and animal sources can cause liver damage and birth defects. Instead, she can get her vitamin A by eating produce such as carrots, broccoli, squash, spinach, kale, and sweet potatoes, which contain beta-carotene, a substance the body can convert to vitamin A. Rule of thumb: stick with one prenatal vitamin a day, and have your woman check with her doctor or registered dietician before adding other vitamins to the mix.

VITAMIN A. It promotes healthy skin, good eyesight, and bone and tooth growth in the fetus. Sources include carrots, dark leafy greens, cantaloupe, and apricots.

VITAMIN C. For the baby, it promotes formation of healthy bones, teeth, and gums while helping the expectant mom with iron absorption. It also makes the body more resistant to infection. Sources include citrus fruits, broccoli, tomatoes, peppers, and potatoes.

A balanced prenatal diet also should include healthy amounts of magnesium, zinc, phosphorus, thiamin (vitamin B1), riboflavin (vitamin B2), vitamins B6 and B12, vitamins D and E, and niacin.

HANDLE WITH CARE

As the pregnant woman's occasional cook and manservant, serving nutritious foods is a powerful way to ensure she and the baby are at their healthiest. But that's just part of the health equation. You need to follow safe food handling procedures. Failing to do so could expose your woman to harmful, illness-causing bacteria, which can land her at the doctor's office and you, the culpable cook, in the doghouse.

So when you are working in the kitchen, help prevent food-borne illness by ensuring you:

DEFREEZE IT RIGHT. Defrost food in the refrigerator or under cold running water. Never let food thaw at room temperature, and don't leave it to defrost out in the elements like the Neanderthals did. Also, never thaw meat on racks above fresh foods. If meat juice drips onto the fresh foods, they'll be contaminated.

ALWAYS USE CLEAN HANDS. Wash your hands after using the bathroom and wash up after handling raw meat, raw poultry, or raw seafood. Bottom line: wash your hands frequently and dry them with a clean towel.

AVOID CROSS-CONTAMINATION. Raw meat and the juice it produces don't mix well with other ingredients. In fact, the bacteria hiding in some meat can be downright dangerous to a person's health, particularly if that person happens to be pregnant. So if you have cut raw chicken on a cutting board, for example, don't use the same board to cut you're veggies until you have washed it thoroughly. And while you're at it, remember to wash the knife. Likewise, to avoid foodborne illnesses, wash your hands with hot, soapy water before and after handling fresh produce or raw meat, poultry, or seafood, as well as after using the bathroom, changing diapers, or handling pets.

AVOID BUYING PRODUCE THAT IS BRUISED OR DAMAGED. It is more likely to harbor bacteria that may cause a food-borne illness, according to the U.S. Food and Drug Administration. If buying fresh-cut produce, be sure it is refrigerated or surrounded by ice. Fresh produce should be refrigerated within two hours of peeling or cutting, according to the FDA, while leftover cut produce should be discarded if left at room temperature for more than two hours.

WASH ALL PRODUCE. Don't let the beautiful shine to those apples fool you. Growers often treat fruits and vegetables with substances that protect them from the elements and pests, so when they arrive in the store they look fresh and appealing to the shopper. Not only may produce be treated with pesticides and fungicides that aren't particularly healthy for a pregnant woman—or anyone else—to ingest, but it also is subject to quite a bit of handling before it reaches your wheeled chariot. Consuming unwashed produce also increases the risk of contracting a food-borne illness. So whether you gathered them from a supermarket, specialty grocer, or produce stand, most fruits and vegetables you buy should be washed thoroughly with cool tap water (no soap, however) or scrubbed before you eat or cook with them, according to the FDA. The exception is produce that will be peeled or skinned before eating—items such as bananas, corn on the cob, onions, and melon whose outer layer typically is not eaten (except by women with Pica, see p. 123).

COOK TO DONENESS. We hate to advocate overcooking a piece of meat that tastes best when it's medium-rare, but during pregnancy, it's best to err on the side of caution by cooking meats that will be served to a pregnant woman more than you might otherwise. The primary reason for caution is

COOKIN' FOR THE PREGNANT BELLY WITH KELLI

PASS ON BRIE, PASS THE PASTEURIZED CHEESELIKE SUBSTANCE

You would rather indulge the pregnant lady in your life than deprive her of some of her favorite food items. But there are some things she absolutely should not eat during pregnancy because of the potential health risks they pose to her and the baby. Foods to avoid include:

- Unpasteurized milk
- Hot dogs and luncheon meats, unless recooked until steaming hot
- Unpasteurized (soft) cheeses such as Brie, Camembert, unpasteurized feta, blue-veined cheeses, and the Mexican fresh cheeses queso fresco and asadero
- Undercooked or uncooked meat, fish (such as sushi), and shellfish
- Uncooked eggs
- Refrigerated pâtés and cheese spreads
- Refrigerated, smoked seafood (canned is OK)
- Unpasteurized juice and cider (to avoid salmonellosis)
- Alfalfa sprouts

a nasty little parasite named *Toxoplasma gondii* that is often present in raw or undercooked meat (and cat feces, as you learned in Chapter 3). Approximately 40 percent of pregnant women who contract the parasite pass it on to their fetus, which raises the risk of mental retardation and miscarriage. That risk is reason enough to be extra careful with your lady's food—and remember, you can always pull your own portion off the fire early if it better suits your Neanderthal tastes. Also keep in mind that even if for safety's sake you need to cook something longer than you'd prefer, you can always add flavor and moisture by accompanying the dish with a superb sauce.

So how to tell if meat is done enough for a pregnant woman? **Chicken** and **turkey** are ready when they are completely cooked through, with their juice running clear and no trace of pink. With a meat thermometer at the ready, cook white meat to 170°F and dark meat to 180°F. **Fish** should be cooked all the way through until it flakes when a fork is inserted. **Pork** and **beef** should be cooked to an internal temperature of 155°F to 165°F. Here it's worth noting that the temperature of cooked foods increases by about 10° after it has been removed from heat. So let meat "rest" for five to ten minutes to allow cooking to finish and for juices to be properly reabsorbed in the meat.

BEWARE OF LISTERIOSIS. Here's another exotic illness you probably have never heard of. It's food-borne and caused by bacteria found in soil and water. One-third of all listeriosis cases occur in pregnant women, so it's not something to be ignored. Listeriosis bacteria are most often found in soft cheeses, undercooked chicken and uncooked hot dogs (see "Cookin' for the Pregnant Belly With Kelli," p. 130). Listeria bacteria are tough little buggers, resistant to heat and many common preservatives. The consequences of listeriosis can be severe, including premature delivery, infection of the newborn, and stillbirth.

MAKING SENSE OF THE RECIPES

Expectant parents tend to be busy folks, with little patience for following intricate, time-consuming recipes. When it comes to kitchen activities, expectant cavemen may be not only short on time and patience, they also are likely working with a deficit of skill and knowledge.

But armed with a few essential tools, ingredients, and techniques, even a caveman with embryonic kitchen skills can overcome his limitations if the recipes he's cooking are simple and the results they produce are satisfying. Cavemen tend to be adventurous creatures. Thus, many of the recipes in this chapter encourage the cook to be curious, courageous, and creative investigating ingredient substitutes and additions. We not only recommend, we demand that you experiment with and deviate from these

PONDER THIS

FISH ARE FINE— JUST THROW BACK THE BIG ONES

One reason Cro-Magnons outlived Neanderthals is because they ate a diet that included fish, which are low in unhealthy fats, high in protein, and packed with good omega fatty acids. Before breaking out the fly rod or spear, however, it's important for the caveman to know that certain species of fish and aquatic life contain high levels of environmental toxins such as PCBs (polychlorinated biphenyls) and methylmercury that can endanger the health of a developing fetus. Larger species of fish generally live longer, so if they dwell in waters where toxins are present, their exposure to those toxins tends to be greater. The U.S. Food and Drug Administration suggests that pregnant women (and women who may become pregnant) avoid consumption of large fish. Avoid shark, swordfish, king mackerel, and tilefish because they may contain high levels of mercury, which can harm the developing nervous system of an unborn baby. According to the FDA, it's fine for pregnant women to eat a variety of fish and shellfish, with a concentration on smaller species and a limit of twelve ounces (about two servings) of fish per week. The agency mentions shrimp, canned light tuna, salmon, pollock, and catfish as being low in mercury. Albacore tuna tends to have more mercury than canned light tuna, so the FDA recommends pregnant women eat no more than one six ounce helping of it per week. For more information, visit the agency's seafood safety website at www.cfsan.fda.gov/seafood1.html.

RECIPE RATING SYSTEM

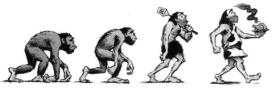

Recipes labeled with a Knuckledragger are the easiest to prepare. At the other end of the spectrum, those labeled with the fully upright Homo sapiens *character are the most advanced—though still relatively simple and quick to make.*

The following profiles can help determine where your culinary skills fall on the spectrum:

The **KNUCKLEDRAGGER** *is what his name implies, someone whose hands have been used mainly for personal propulsion and a bit of grooming but almost never for food preparation. He's an absolute beginner in the kitchen.*

The more evolved but still very primitive **NEANDERTHAL** *has a limited grasp of kitchen tools and food preparation but needs lots of help to overcome his culinary clumsiness.*

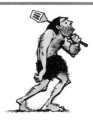

HOMO HABILIS (HANDY MAN) *represents a male who, with a little more polish and seasoning, is on his way to being fully self-sufficient in the kitchen.*

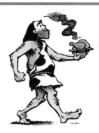

By the time your baby comes, the hope is you'll have the skills to join the elite **HOMO SAPIENS** *group at the top of the evolutionary heap. The* Homo sapiens *depicts a guy who's learned to stand on his own as a cook, who's fully able to gather all ingredients and cook them properly so he can bask in the glory of a grateful family.*

recipes if you see fit in order to stumble upon your own signature creations. Many of the recipes also have leftover potential, because as anyone who has been through pregnancy and parenthood knows, homemade leftovers are great to have on standby in the fridge or freezer for an easy, healthy meal anytime.

We've noticeably omitted recipes for breads and desserts because, in our humble opinion, your time would be better spent on other activities. It can be messy and time-consuming to make a dessert, so we recommend leaving it to the pros. Give your quality corner bakery some business and you will free up much needed time, as well as end up eating a better product.

Before you strap on the apron and start cooking, here's a quick primer on how the recipes that follow are rated and structured:

DEGREE OF DIFFICULTY. It took our ancestors millions of years to harness the power of fire, to develop tools and weapons for capturing and slaughtering prey (food), and to figure out how to prepare and cook whatever they managed to drag back to the cave. Our caveman ancestors needed hundreds of generations to get the cooking thing down, so don't expect to become an overnight sensation in the kitchen. You have to walk upright before you can run.

Rather than rush the evolutionary process, the recipes included in this book nurture it. Each recipe is rated on a scale of simplicity represented by four caveman characters. The more upright the character, the more "evolved" the recipe.

TOOLS OF THE TRADE

If your knowledge of kitchen instruments starts and ends with the knife, spoon, and fork, here are some additional items you may want to have around as you launch your caveman cooking career.

SPATULA Here's a less hazardous, more hygienic alternative to flipping hot items with callused hands.

MEASURING SPOONS, MEASURING CUP(S) These may not be necessary for the firepit cooking you know and love, but when you come in from the cold, "eyeballing" ingredients will only get you in trouble.

MEAT THERMOMETER Tests the proper cooked interior temperature of meats

FOOD PROCESSOR It slices, it dices! This timesaving device also may save a trip or two to the hospital emergency room until your knife skills evolve.

BASTING BRUSH An essential tool for lathering meats with sauces

WIRE RACK Great for the oven or the countertop for cooling

GRILLING SCREENS (see p. 142)

ROLLING PIN Excellent cudgel or prep tool for dough

COLANDER For straining pasta, stovetop steaming, or washing vegetables in the sink

HAIRNET For the follicly well-endowed members of the species who are more apt to shed

OVEN MITT(S) Your calluses are tough but they're not coated with asbestos, so you'll need mitts (or a folded kitchen towel) to hold hot pans.

TONGS A key defense against having to reach into boiling water and the heart of a flame

WIRE WHISK Nice for combining wet and dry ingredients

ELECTRIC MIXER Ultimate tool for mocktails (for her) and cocktails (for you) and smoothies (for both of you)

A SET OF QUALITY KNIVES May already be part of your hunting arsenal

SPRAY BOTTLE Excellent BBQ tool for controlling flames and/or keeping meats moist

SKEWERS Wood or metal grilling tool for the BBQ

NONSTICK SKILLET/PANS These are essential to cooking many breakfast items, including the "world's fluffiest pancake" recipe provided here. Most importantly, they are easy to clean.

GARLIC PRESS Fast crushing tool for the "stinking rose"

APRON To protect your animal pelt wardrobe

SHEET PANS Metal cookie-type sheet for the oven.

CUTTING BOARD(S) Preserve countertops with cutting boards, and remember to clean them thoroughly after cutting potential bacteria-carrying items such as raw meat.

IMMERSION BLENDER A.K.A. stick blender or "boat motor" for mixing soups and sauces, or making smoothies

MEASUREMENTS AND CONVERSIONS

BASIC U.S. MEASUREMENTS

1 tablespoon (tbsp) =
3 teaspoons (tsp) = 1/16 cup

2 tablespoons = 1/8 cup = 1 ounce (oz)

4 tablespoons = 1/4 cup

5 tablespoons + 1 teaspoon = 1/3 cup

8 tablespoons = 1/2 cup

10 tablespoons + 2 teaspoons = 2/3 cup

12 tablespoons = 3/4 cup

1 cup = 48 teaspoons

1 cup = 16 tablespoons

1 cup = 8 fluid ounces (fl oz)

1 pint (pt) = 2 cups

1 quart (qt) = 2 pints

1 quart = 4 cups

4 quarts = 1 gallon (gal)

16 ounces (oz) = 1 pound (lb)

U.S. TO METRIC CONVERSIONS

1 teaspoon = 5 ml

1 tablespoon = 15 ml

1 fluid oz = 30 ml

1 cup = 237 ml

2 cups (1 pint) = 473 ml

4 cups (1 quart) = 0.95 liter

1 quart = 0.946 liters

4 quarts (1 gallon) = 3.8 liters

1 oz = 28 grams

1 lb = 454 grams

1 lb = 0.454 kilograms

Cooking temperature:
to convert Fahrenheit (F)
to Celsius (C): $0.555 \times (°F - 32)$

METRIC TO U.S. CONVERSIONS

1 milliliter = 1/5 teaspoon

100 ml = 3.4 fluid oz

1 liter = 34 fluid oz =
4.2 cups = 2.1 pints =
1.06 quarts = 0.26 gallon

1 gram = 0.035 ounce

1 kilogram = 2.205 lb = 35 ounces

1 kilogram = 2.205 pounds

Cooking temperature:
to convert Celsius to Fahrenheit:
$1.8 \times (°C + 32)$

1 milliliter (ml) =
1 cubic centimeter (cc)

Source: United States Dept. of Agriculture (USDA)

COOKING BY THE NUMBERS. For the Cro-Magnons of the Paleolithic period, a cave dwelling not only provided shelter for the clan and their animals, it also may have doubled as a one-room schoolhouse. It could have been a place where elder clan members educated their young, passing on knowledge, techniques, and customs important to the survival of the species and its culture. It may also have been where Cro-Magnon youth learned how to build a fire and butcher a goat, how to whittle an arrow and sharpen a spear, how to distinguish between edible and nonedible nuts, berries, and mushrooms and, of course, how to transform the ingredients they hunted and gathered into a palatable meal.

Passing cooking methods down from one caveman generation to the next required a grasp of basic measurement factors as well as rudimentary mathematic skills. How many pinches to a fistful? How many fistfuls make a bunch? How many bunches in a bushel? Learning these basic units may have helped the Cro-Magnon pass on recipes. But when measurements units and techniques differed from cave to cave, it made interclan recipe sharing difficult.

Similar differences in measurement units and technique exist even today. There's the clan that sticks to metric measurements, then there's the clan that relies on standard or u.s. measurements. It's helpful for the modern caveman cook to be able to convert between the two. Here, then, is a handy conversion chart to allow even the thickest-skulled males to make easy conversions.

RISE AND DINE

I went to a café that advertised "breakfast anytime," so I ordered french toast during the Renaissance.
—STEPHEN WRIGHT

What's not to love about breakfast? Usually with a minimum of effort, the caveman can produce a nutritious, tasteful *petite dejeuner* and earn major kudos from his woman in the process. By rising early and letting your lady sleep while you cook, you could put yourself in position to be on the golf course or chasing down a mastodon by mid-morning.

Your first job is to ensure that your lady's daily nutritional and caloric requirements are met, so for her (and for a healthy you), skipping breakfast is out of the question. Your woman's body has been busy overnight supplying nutrition to the growing baby, so she may not have absorbed enough nutrients for herself, which means her body is in need of replenishment in the morning.

Here's your chance to embrace the sunrise, prepare some good coffee (if she's drinking caffeinated beverages during pregnancy), even squeeze some fresh orange juice, and enjoy cooking a meal that is prepared to your woman's tastes. Your effort should earn you great appreciation and perhaps some weekend freedom when the golf course, river, or shooting range beckons.

The breakfast recipes provided here all work well as leftovers. Make extra on a weekend morning and you'll rest easy knowing you'll have access to breakfast leftovers to meet her nutritional needs later in the week.

THE WORLD'S BEST FLUFFY PANCAKES

SERVES: two to four

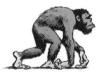

RATING: Knuckledragger

ESTIMATED PREP AND COOKING TIME:
thirty minutes

TOOLS: fork, two bowls, whisk, nonstick skillet, brush, spatula, knife

NEED FIRE? yes, from a stovetop burner (gas or electric)

GATHER:

1 cup	all-purpose flour (or wheat for added fiber)
1 tbsp	sugar
1 tbsp	baking powder
¼ tsp	baking soda
¼ tsp	salt
1	egg
1 cup	milk
1 (8 oz)	container of yogurt
	maple syrup
	fresh sliced fruit (optional)
	wheat germ (optional)

These terrific pancakes beat any made from premixed batter. They are even better with fresh, sliced fruit. For example, thinly slice a banana and add it to the top of the batter when it is poured onto the skillet. When the pancake is flipped and finished with the banana side down, the sugars in the fruit caramelize with perfect results.

You can also top pancakes with wheat germ for great crunch, flavor, and added health benefits.

DIRECTIONS:

➤ In a medium bowl, combine dry ingredients (flour, sugar, baking powder, baking soda, salt) and mix well.

➤ In a separate bowl, whisk eggs until well beaten and add milk and yogurt until smooth.

➤ Make a well in the center of the dry ingredients.

➤ Pour egg mixture in the center and stir just until flour mixture is moistened and incorporated.

➤ Do not overstir; a lumpy mix is perfect for a fluffy pancake.

➤ Preheat a nonstick skillet over medium-high heat and brush with a little vegetable oil to coat.

➤ Pour a quarter cup of batter into skillet and cook until bubbles form on top and the underside is golden brown.

➤ Flip the pancake and cook until second side is golden brown (about two or three minutes).

BREAKFAST STRATA

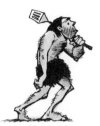

SERVES: two, plus leftovers

RATING: *Homo habilis*

ESTIMATED PREP AND COOKING TIME:
one hour forty-five minutes

TOOLS: casserole/baking dish, food processor, medium saucepan, whisk

NEED FIRE? yes, from an oven

HUNT:

8 oz	crumbled breakfast sausage

GATHER:

1 loaf	thinly sliced Italian bread (stale or lightly toasted)
1	large onion, diced
3 tbsp	unsalted butter
8 oz	white button mushrooms, sliced
8 oz	sundried tomato cream cheese (see right)
6	large eggs
1 ¾ cups	half-and-half
2 cups	baby spinach, loosely packed
	fresh parsley, minced

This is a layered casserole that includes bread, eggs, cheese, and cream. As he evolves, the creative caveman cook can substitute and add ingredients to this basic strata recipe. The most important thing to keep in mind when adding different ingredients is to control overall water content. Moisture-laden additions (such as undrained tomatoes) can turn this dish to mush, threatening the integrity of the strata you have worked so hard to assemble. Strata should have discernible layers, so avoid the temptation to overload with ingredients. Using a minimalist approach with quality ingredients greatly increases the odds for successful stratification. Because this is a layered dish, use thin slices of stale bread. If you don't have stale Italian bread lying around, substitute bread slices lightly toasted in the oven before assembly.

SUNDRIED TOMATO CREAM CHEESE

In a food processor, mix cream cheese, four ounces sundried tomato in oil (the amount typically found in a small, store-bought jar), drained, salted, and peppered (with freshly ground pepper) to taste. Push the button and you have a great addition to many savory meals. Like compound butters (see flank steak recipe), cream cheese is a sponge for absorbing flavors. A few items to experiment with include fresh herbs, roasted garlic, avocado, nuts, and a lime/jalapeño combination.

TO ASSEMBLE STRATA:

▶ Heat two tablespoons of butter in a medium saucepan.

▶ Add onion, sausage, and mushroom, and sauté until sausage is cooked and onions

are translucent, four to five minutes.
Set aside.

- ▸ Butter an eight-inch square baking dish with the remaining tablespoon of butter.

- ▸ Spread half the sundried tomato cream cheese on bread and arrange in bottom of baking dish.

- ▸ Top the cream cheese with half the sausage mixture and half the baby spinach. Repeat the step by spreading cream cheese on the remaining bread and top with remaining sausage and spinach.

- ▸ Whisk the eggs and half-and-half together.

- ▸ Add salt and freshly ground pepper to taste.

- ▸ Pour the egg mixture evenly over the bread layers and cover the surface with plastic wrap.

- ▸ Refrigerate for one hour or overnight.

- ▸ Preheat oven to 325°.

- ▸ Bake until the center of the strata is puffed and the edges of the strata have pulled slightly away from the baking dish, usually fifty minutes to one hour.

- ▸ Cool on a wire rack before serving.

PONDER THIS

PORK-O-RAMA

Ever had the urge to cook a whole pound of bacon at once but lacked a surface large enough to do so? Here is your answer. Put a wire rack on a baking sheet/pan and cook bacon (or sausage) in the oven at 350° for a relatively mess-free experience. This method frees time and space on the stove to cook pancakes. These handy pans also work great to keep breakfast items warm in the oven while you finish cooking and cleaning.

PONDER THIS

EGG-CELLENT SCRAMBLERS

When cooking scrambled eggs, whisk a little half-and-half into the eggs and cook over low heat, stirring frequently, for creamy and great-tasting results. Also add a cream cheese compound for added richness and flavor.

HOMEMADE GRANOLA WITH YOGURT AND FRESH FRUIT

SERVES: six to eight

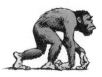

RATING: Knuckledragger

ESTIMATED PREP AND COOKING TIME:
thirty minutes

TOOLS: measuring cups, saucepan, two baking sheets, large bowl, fork

NEED FIRE? yes, from an oven

GATHER:

8 cups	rolled oats
½ cup	vegetable oil
½ cup	brown sugar (to taste)
1 cup	honey
1 tsp	pure vanilla extract
1 tbsp	ground cinnamon, or to taste
¼ tsp	salt
2 cups	sunflower seeds
1 ½ cups	slivered almonds
2 cups	raisins or dried cherries
1 cup	dried apricot, chopped

For our caveman ancestors, nuts and berries were like meat and potatoes are today. Now those same ingredients can be transformed into a hearty and healthful granola that can be eaten at breakfast or during hungry moments throughout the day. Make enough and keep it in an airtight container—granola stays fresh and tasty for a week or more. Homemade granola is far more tasty and better for mom than the supersweet versions found in supermarkets.

DIRECTIONS:

➤ Preheat the oven to 350°.

➤ In a medium saucepan, heat oil, brown sugar, honey, vanilla, cinnamon, and salt over medium heat until the brown sugar has incorporated (melted into other ingredients), about five minutes.

➤ In a large bowl, mix oatmeal, sunflower seeds, and almonds.

➤ Pour the oil mixture over the oatmeal and toss to combine.

➤ Spread evenly over two baking sheets and bake for fifteen minutes (stir once at the ten-minute mark).

➤ Combine dried fruit after the granola is cooked.

➤ Serve with yogurt and fresh fruit of your choice.

PSYCHO GRILLER: RECIPES FOR THE BARBEQUE

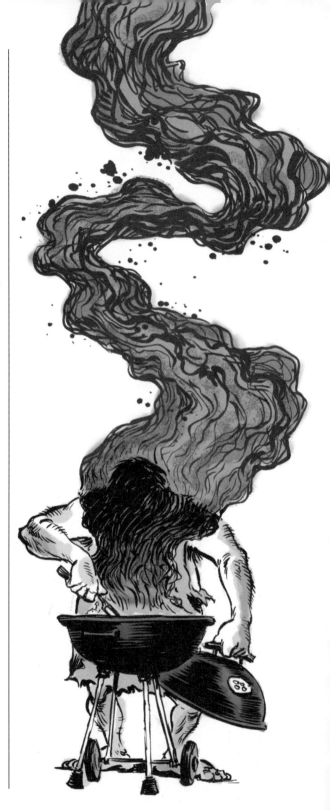

No time to wallow in the mire
C'mon baby light my fire

—THE DOORS, "LIGHT MY FIRE"

The ultimate form of caveman cooking, the technique nearest and dearest to our hearts, is grilling over flame. Even the father of classical cuisine, Auguste Escoffier, traced all cooking back to our caveman brethren when he described grilling as "the remote starting point, the very genesis of our art." Nothing beats heading outdoors, opening a cold beer, and smelling the sweet aroma of searing flesh on the fire. There is a right way to do it, and we're here to tell you how it's done.

One of the best things you can do to evolve into a grilling maestro is to get to know your local butcher. If ever a man has earned the right to be called a throwback, it is the butcher, who has chosen to spend most of his waking hours in hip boots, armed with an array of knives and saws, hacking meat apart in a freezing-cold vault. In a long-ago era his clan probably would have made him chieftain or king due to his prowess with all types of handheld weaponry. But nowadays he is behind the counter at a shop or supermarket, waiting to discuss the subtleties of connective tissues in various cuts of meats. He has the tools and experience to make your job easier and more enjoyable by choosing for you the perfect cuts for any need or recipe and then trimming them to perfection. A good butcher is every bit as important in your life as a good buddy, barber, or bookie.

Whether you're into charcoal or gas, there are some ground rules to follow before starting. First, any grill should be cleaned and preheated to achieve desired results. A true culinary caveman loves a hot grill. A hot grill is one that when you hold your hand three inches over the cooking surface, it takes about three seconds before a blood-curdling scream frightens the neighborhood.

You can grill directly over a hot flame (direct heat) or you can cook over a cooler portion of the grill with the lid closed, creating more of an oven effect (indirect heat). Because thoroughly cooking food for a pregnant woman is a top priority, more often than not you will be using some indirect heat while grilling. There is a highly recommended happy medium between the two types of grilling: sear the meat—or whatever protein you're cooking—directly on the hottest part of the grill, creating a wonderful and flavorful crust, then finish the cooking process indirectly over one of the grill's cooler zones with a closed lid. Everyone is happy because you get to beat your chest and chant at the flames while searing your chops, and she can enjoy her meal knowing you have cooked the food in a safe manner.

While cooking a piece of meat to 170° makes many a bloodthirsty, I-like-my-meat-still-mooing caveman cringe, your lady will appreciate your thoughtfulness. To keep the meat fairly tender, use the direct heat sear and the indirect finish method, then make a nice sauce to accompany your carcass of choice. You can always order that "blue" steak when you go out to eat.

Word to the wise griller: if you have some extra time, it's worth buying a larger cut of meat and cooking it "low and slow" (low temperature, long cooking time), which breaks down the meat's connective tissue, making it more tender.

GRILLING NECESSITIES

Chances are you already have a fairly impressive array of grilling tools. Here are some that all cavemen should have in their collection:

▶ **THERMOMETER,** preferably instant-read. The most important tool for our most important rule: Do No Harm. Poking and prodding cooking meat with your hairy fingers to test doneness might work around the open firepit, but it certainly won't fly when cooking for a pregnant woman. You must be sure the protein you are cooking (particularly chicken, pork, and ground beef) is heated to a temperature that is high enough to kill any parasites. The only way to be sure meat is safe to eat is to either cook it until it has the taste and texture of a hockey puck or to use a thermometer.

▶ **SPATULA, TONGS:** Not only do these make engaging playthings for the cavetot, they also are indispensable grilling tools. Look for quality, stainless steel varieties that stand the test of time. Spatulas are practical to help with meat that sticks to the grill and to move smaller cuts of meat and fish. Tongs are useful in placing foods such as ribs, chicken, and sausage on the grill and in rearranging hot coals in the fire.

▶ **BASTING BRUSHES:** Use brushes to apply sauces during grilling. Take care not to add sugary glazes like BBQ sauces until the very end of cooking to avoid burning.

▶ **SKEWERS:** Accomplished grill jockeys prefer flat-edge metal skewers that help prevent the food on a kebab from turning on the grill. If you have wooden skewers, soak them in water prior to use so they don't catch fire on the grill.

▶ **GRILL SCREENS:** Use these to prevent retrieval burns when shrimp, vegetables, or other items slip through the cracks. They also work great for cooking pizza on the grill (a recipe for grilled pizza comes later in this chapter). Remember to brush the screen with oil and let it preheat before adding food.

▶ **SPRAY BOTTLES:** The smart caveman cook is prepared for anything, so he keeps a fire extinguisher indoors, in or near the kitchen, and a spray bottle full of water next to his charcoal grill to douse a flame that's too high. You can also fill a spray bottle with apple juice or citrus juice to spray on your food while it's grilling to add additional flavor and moistness.

PONDER THIS

HIGH-TOUCH MEALS

When the stress of pregnancy mounts and the two of you crave romance, it's time for the caveman to turn on the charm by surprising his woman with breakfast in bed or a candlelight dinner. It doesn't take much on the breakfast side: make sure your woman stays in bed while you put together a meal that includes entrée, fresh-squeezed juice and/or coffee, a side such as fresh fruit, utensils, and a napkin. Load it all on a tray, add a vase with a freshly cut flower, and carefully tote it to the bedroom. For dinner, it's all about ambience. Light candles, set the table with your fine silver, put on some background mood music (or hire a strolling minstrel), dim the overhead lights, pour two glasses of wine (hers can be sparkling cider or a nonalcoholic wine), and pull out her chair when she's ready to be seated. Then bring courses out from the kitchen one by one, concluding with a fancy dessert (furnished by your friend the corner baker).

SOUTHWEST FLANK STEAK WITH CILANTRO BUTTER

This recipe addresses three important cooking topics:

- how to properly grill a steak;

- how to use spice rubs; and

- how to make a compound butter to liven up a dish.

Why do you think simple dishes such as steak often taste better at good restaurants than at home? It's basically the same cut of meat you use at home, cooked over a similar flame, so it shouldn't be so different, right?

The major distinction is that most home cooks underseason meat. Adding a bit of salt doesn't quite cut it. No, you need proper and bold seasoning when grilling. That's where spice rubs come in. Whether it's an Indian, Thai, French, Southwestern, or Cro-Magnon meal, a good rub can improve it. Keep in mind that any dry spice rub can also be made into a paste by adding olive oil, garlic, and fresh herbs.

BASIC SOUTHWESTERN SPICE RUB

Mix all ingredients together in a small bowl. Now you have a dry spice rub you can use right away or keep for several weeks in an airtight container.

(continued on next page)

SERVES: two to four
(fewer eaters means more leftovers)

RATING: Neanderthal

ESTIMATED PREP AND COOKING TIME: thirty-five minutes

TOOLS: bowl, mixing utensil such as a fork, measuring spoon, tongs, plastic wrap, chopping knife

NEED FIRE? yes, grill

HUNT:

1¼–1½ lbs	flank steak

GATHER:

BASIC SOUTHWESTERN SPICE RUB:

2 tbsp	salt
2 tbsp	paprika
2 tbsp	ground cumin
2 tbsp	chili powder
1 tbsp	ground black pepper
1 tbsp	dried oregano
1 tsp	sugar
1–2 tsp	cayenne pepper

COMPOUND BUTTER

4 oz	butter (full stick or less will do) leave it out for 30 minutes or so to soften
1 small bunch	cilantro, finely chopped

COMPOUND BUTTER

Butter has a nice flavor on its own. What's more, the fat it contains creates a wonderful sponge effect, allowing it to absorb other flavorful ingredients. Butter with added ingredients is called a compound butter. To make one:

▶ Finely chop a tablespoon or two of your chosen ingredient(s)—fresh herbs, garlic, horseradish, or wasabi (which may be too hot for a pregnant woman's taste; ask her), hot chiles, ginger, citrus, or balsamic vinegar

▶ Put it in a bowl with a stick of butter and mash it all together with a fork, adding salt and pepper to taste.

▶ Roll the butter in plastic wrap into a small log and refrigerate.

The butter can be refrigerated for up to a week or frozen for many weeks. Refrigerated butter melts perfectly on hot food, but the frozen variety should be thawed before use.

THE STEAK

A thin cut of meat works well for grilling in general and for Southwestern or Mexican style meals in particular. A long, thin cut can also be cut in half before grilling, so you can pull your piece off when it's cooked to your liking, leaving her piece on until it hits pregnant-lady temp (at least 155°). But before you get cooking:

▶ Liberally season the steaks with the spice rub and refrigerate for one to two hours.

▶ Place the steaks on a hot, clean grill.

▶ After two minutes, give the steaks a quarter-turn (rotating, not flipping), to give them nifty-looking crosshatches.

▶ Turn the steak, and after two minutes, rotate it another quarter-turn.

▶ Cook for two more minutes.

▶ Now the caveman's steak should be cooked to medium-rare; let her steak finish cooking over indirect heat on a cooler part of the grill.

▶ Top the steak with slices of cilantro butter, then cut steak in thin slices, against the grain, to serve.

SHRIMP AND VEGETABLE KEBABS WITH LEMON

SERVES: two to four
(fewer eaters means more leftovers)

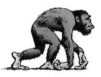

RATING: Knuckledragger

ESTIMATED PREP AND COOKING TIME:
thirty minutes, plus one hour for marination

TOOLS: whisk, skewers (wooden or metal),
medium-size bowl, quality chef's knife,
measuring cup

NEED FIRE? yes, grill

HUNT:

1 lb jumbo shrimp, peeled and deveined

GATHER:

½ cup olive oil

¼ cup dry white wine (substitute 2 tbsp balsamic
vinegar or lemon juice if your woman is
abstaining from alcohol)

1 tbsp fresh thyme, chopped

½ lb white button mushrooms, whole

2 red bell peppers, cut into one-inch squares
for skewering

1 red onion, cut into one-inch wedges for
skewering

salt and black pepper to taste

It doesn't get more primitive than putting your food on sticks and cooking it over a flame. Kebabs are a classic and remain one of the best ways to exhibit your grilling prowess. The beauty of the kebob lies in its simplicity: a complete and nutritious meal supplied on sticks with little mess and great presentation—truly a win-win-win proposition. What's more, the infinite ingredient and marinade possibilities make playing with sticks and fire a safe but sporting activity.

▷ Cut the lemon into small slices, about one-eighth-inch thick.

▷ In a medium bowl, whisk together olive oil, wine, chopped thyme, salt, and pepper.

▷ Add the shrimp, lemons, and vegetables to coat evenly and marinate for up to one hour.

The act of marinating food is a joy for caveman types because it actually is a passive activity that allows a guy to grab a tasty beverage, sit back and relax while the marinade works its magic. Cavemen like slow-cooking turkeys for the same reason.

▷ Skewer shrimp, lemon, and vegetables, alternating to enhance color and presentation. To skewer the shrimp, thread skewer through the tail then add a lemon slice, then bend the shrimp and skewer the top, pinching the lemon between each shrimp.

▷ Preheat the grill and break out the grill rack if you have one. If not, be careful when turning the kebabs, because shrimp can stick and items can be irretrievably lost through the bars of the grill.

- Arrange the skewers on the grill rack over direct heat and brush remaining liquid on the kebabs.

- Turn the skewers a couple times to cook evenly. Remove after eight to ten minutes.

Kebabs can be served with any starch—potato, rice, etc.—but a bed of couscous is perfect for this Mediterranean meal.

Couscous is a fine-grained, easy-to-prepare pasta you can buy in bulk or by the box at your local supermarket or specialty store. To cook, follow the instructions on the package.

GRILLED PIZZA

SERVES: six to eight

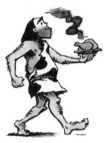

RATING: *Homo sapiens*

ESTIMATED PREP AND COOKING TIME: one hour, plus one and a half to two hours for dough to rise (watching dough rise—now that's a caveman's kind of work!)

TOOLS: food processor, measuring spoons/cups, plastic wrap, rolling pin, spatula(s) for removing pizza from grill

NEED FIRE? yes, grill

HUNT:

meat of choice (sausage, pepperoni, dried mastodon, etc.)

GATHER:

FOR THE DOUGH:

2 tbsp	extra virgin olive oil
1 cup	water, room temperature
2 cups	flour, plus more for the work surface
2 tsp	sugar
1 tsp	salt
1 tsp	fast-acting yeast
	parchment or waxed paper
	nonstick cooking spray

1	chopped or sliced tomato (medium to large)
3–4 oz	cheese (fresh mozzarella for a classic pizza)
2 tbsp	fresh, finely chopped herbs (basil and oregano are excellent on pizza)
1–2 cloves	fresh or roasted garlic, finely chopped or pressed

Grilled pizza? Say what? When you first tell your lady you plan to grill a pizza for dinner, she may be skeptical, assuming you're merely making a sad excuse to get into that cooler full of beer you have stashed under the deck. However, the beer stash is just a fringe benefit to what could quickly become a staple in your culinary arsenal. The trick to any good pizza is a great crust, and this version is guaranteed not to disappoint.

Remember that quality ingredients, not heaping quantities, are what make this pizza outstanding. The list of toppings for this pizza is as boundless as your imagination, so have fun and experiment, remembering not to use ingredients that offend the pregnant woman's senses.

Include as many veggies as possible for a healthy and delicious pizza that is nutritious for the apple of your eye.

This grilled crust also works great for a dessert pizza topped with chocolate and fresh fruit or cinnamon and honey.

PIZZA DOUGH

➤ Place the dry ingredients (flour, sugar, salt, yeast) in a food processor and press the "pulse" button to blend them.

➤ Combine oil and water, and with the food processor running slowly, add liquid to the dry ingredients until a ball is formed.

➤ Spray a glass bowl with nonstick cooking spray and press the ball of dough inside the bowl so it is flat on top.

➤ Cover with plastic wrap until it doubles in size, approximately two hours.

➤ When dough has doubled in size, cut it in half, then cut each piece in half again so you have four pieces.

➤ Form each piece into a smooth ball and on a clean, floured surface, roll the dough into thin roundish shapes, eight to nine inches in diameter.

Don't worry about making them perfectly circular. You're not inventing the wheel yet, caveman. Strange shapes have a primitive, rough-hewn quality, and they will taste just as good as a pie that's perfectly round.

➤ Place on floured parchment paper.

This recipe is for four pizza crusts, so if one pizza is enough, wrap the other dough balls in plastic wrap and refrigerate or freeze for later use.

➤ Transfer dough rounds from floured parchment paper to a preheated, medium-hot grill.

▶ Keep your eye on the crust because it doesn't take long to cook (two minutes or so usually). It's good to have a small amount of char on the pizza to ensure that it will be crispy.

Pull the crust off the fire carefully and transfer it indoors to a clean work surface, browned side up. Apply toppings to the browned side, then return the topped pie to the grill, cooking it until the cheese has melted and the bottom has browned.

GRILLED PIZZA TOPPINGS

The key to this pizza is its lack of traditional sauce toppings. A wet sauce only defeats the purpose of this great crunchy-style pizza. Instead, you will use diced or sliced tomatoes, quality extra virgin olive oil, fresh herbs, and quality cheese. This combination will reward you with some of the best pizza you've ever tasted.

ONE-POT WONDERS

A blazing, log-stoked fire laps the edge of the broad metal cauldron suspended above the flames, causing a pungent steam to rise to the dark heights of the cavernous ceiling overhead. A man clad in pelts and worn leather catapults large pieces of vegetation and unidentifiable cuts of meat into the dark, roiling waters, occasionally stirring the contents with a large wooden utensil. For the prehistoric people who live here and for the bats that hang unseen above them, it's another aromatic evening of one-pot meal-making, Bronze Age style.

From pasta dishes to stew, risotto, soups, and beyond, one-pot meals remain a staple of mankind's menu. They are especially beloved by the omnivorous cavemen that walk among us today for the simplicity, convenience, and multiple-helping satisfaction they provide. For the expectant couple, they make a straightforward, splendid meal to enjoy now or to save in the freezer for reheating after the baby has been born, when time and parental energy levels are especially low.

Preparing one-pot meals gives the caveman a great chance to apply the Do-No-Harm principles adapted from Hippocrates. A policy in which you clean, dry, and put away items you have used but no longer need to prepare the meal keeps clutter and postmeal cleanup to a minimum. For the caveman, this is one part of life he can control. When other parts of life seem to be spinning out of control, at least he can keep order in the kitchen universe. Thus, the "let it soak" mentality must go.

The idea behind one-pot cooking is appealing in its simplicity: prep multiple ingredients, including meat and/or vegetables, toss them all in the pot with some liquid and some herbs and spices, put the pot over heat for a period of time, then serve the delicious result. If you have people staying at your house before, during, and after the birth, it's always nice to fall back on a one-pot wonder.

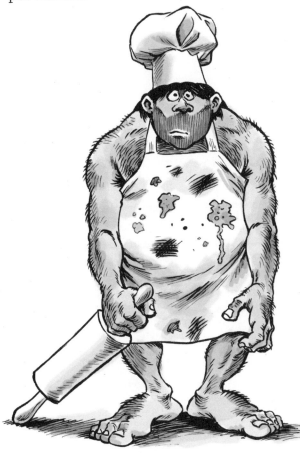

PONDER THIS

A KNACK FOR NOODLES

Pasta dishes should be like an arrow in your culinary quiver or a rock in your gastronomical pouch, always at the ready to satisfy. They meet all the culinary caveman's qualifications: ease of preparation, low-impact on the kitchen, and healthy, with good leftover potential. Although many pasta dishes are simple, most people still find a way to screw them up. The biggest mistake made in pasta preparation is overcooking the noodles in too small a pot. All too frequently the greenhorn caveman creates a starchy, sticky mess. Go for the big pot instead, as you'll need about five quarts of boiling water to give sufficient space for one pound of pasta to circulate within. Measure it out the first time and you'll remember just where to fill the pot. Cooking times for pasta vary according to size, shape, and vintage (fresh pasta cooks much more quickly than dried). To test for doneness, rather than the highly satisfying method of tossing the noodle against a wall to see if it sticks, try the more cultivated approach of removing a small sample, running it under water, and tasting for doneness. Remember, pasta tends to continue cooking even after it is removed from heat, so take it out just before it's perfectly done for you. For baked dishes such as lasagna, undercook the pasta, as it will keep cooking during the baking process.

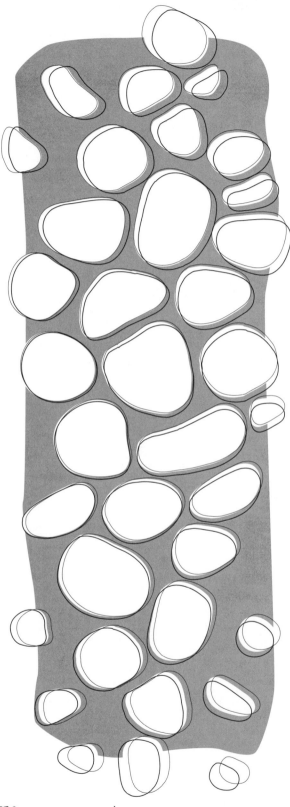

CLASSIC AMERICAN LASAGNA BOLOGNESE

....

Blessed are the cheesemakers

—J. CHRIST, MONTY PYTHON'S *LIFE OF BRIAN*

....

SERVES: six to eight

....

RATING: Neanderthal

....

ESTIMATED PREP AND COOKING TIME:
seventy-five minutes

....

TOOLS: colander, spoon

....

NEED FIRE? yes, oven

....

HUNT:

....

	ground beef or sausage (both optional)

....

GATHER:

....

5 quarts	boiling water, lightly salted
12 oz	dried lasagna noodles
2 cups	mozzarella cheese, shredded
	ricotta cheese filling, see below
	nonstick cooking spray or olive oil
	basic tomato sauce, see below

Lasagna is proof that in cooking, simpler is often better. You take some wide noodles, layer sauce and cheese, bake, and—*voilà!*—you have a basic lasagna. Most important in lasagna preparation is to achieve the proper ratio of sauce and ingredients to noodles. The pasta soaks up quite a bit of liquid during baking, so too little sauce means bone-dry lasagna, whereas too much sauce means a sloppy mess. Generally, strive for a constant proportion of pasta to sauce: one quart of sauce for one pound of pasta. The following is a basic lasagna recipe, but we recommend experimenting with different sauces and ingredients. Lasagnas provide an excellent vehicle to slip in nutritious vegetables to help satisfy the nutritional needs of your partner.

▶ Bring the water to a boil and cook the noodles a few at a time. Remove them before they are done (after about five minutes, still firm) and lay them to drain in a colander.

▶ Preheat the oven to 400°.

▶ Spray the bottom of your lasagna pan with nonstick cooking spray or coat with olive oil. Place a layer of noodles in pan, touching but not overlapping.

▶ Spread one-third of the ricotta mixture, then one-third of the basic tomato sauce, then one-third of the mozzarella cheese on top of the first layer of noodles. Repeat two more times.

▶ Bake for thirty to forty minutes until the lasagna is bubbling in many spots along the edges. Remove from oven and let rest for five to ten minutes.

▶ Cut in apportioned squares and serve.

RICOTTA CHEESE FILLING
Mix the following ingredients:

16 oz	ricotta cheese
½ cup	grated Parmesan cheese
1	egg
¼ cup	minced fresh basil leaves
	salt and pepper to taste

BASIC TOMATO SAUCE
This basic tomato sauce is great with ground beef or Italian sausage; add a half-pound to a pound of each, depending on how carnivorous you and your woman are feeling.

3 tbsp	olive oil
3	cloves garlic, minced
1	small onion, diced
1 can (28 oz)	whole plum tomatoes
	salt and pepper to taste

▶ Sauté the onion and garlic in two tablespoons of olive oil over medium-low heat.

▶ Drain the tomatoes, crush with hands, and add them to onion and garlic.

▶ Cook until the tomatoes break down, about ten minutes.

▶ Stir in remaining tablespoon of oil and add salt and pepper to taste.

RISOTTO WITH CHICKEN, ARTICHOKE, AND BABY SPINACH

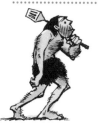

SERVES: four to six

RATING: *Homo habilis*

ESTIMATED PREP AND COOKING TIME:
one hour

TOOLS: medium (2 qt) and large (4 qt) saucepan, measuring cups/spoons, stirring implement, immersion blender (also called a stick blender or "boat motor" in restaurant kitchens, it is invaluable to speed up the process in soup and sauce preparation)

NEED FIRE? yes, stovetop

HUNT: large cooked chicken breast, chopped

GATHER:

6 cups low-sodium chicken broth

4 tbsp unsalted butter

1 medium onion, diced

2 cups arborio rice

1 cup white wine, (optional)

1 cup Parmesan cheese, freshly grated, better-quality (like Parmigiano Reggiano)

1 cup artichoke hearts, sliced

2 cups baby spinach, loosely packed

½ cup pine nuts (pignoli), toasted dry in a sauté pan on the stovetop for 2 to 3 minutes

salt and pepper to taste

When you simmer food, you're using a technique revered by a long line of cavemen cooks. Prehistoric Britons simmered their meat in troughs by adding hot stones from a fire at regular intervals. Then the Bronze Age opened up new possibilities with the arrival of cooking pots that could be held directly over flame. Thus were born soups, stews, and risottos.

Risotto is usually made from arborio rice, an Italian short-grain rice. It is a simple dish that requires a little extra time to make perfect, with a long simmer and lots of stirring. The TLC you provide this dish is well worth it. The rice is the star of risotto, though you can really get creative with the supporting cast—the ingredients you use. Again, the list of possibilities is endless. Once you've learned how to get the proper texture of your rice, these dishes will provide enjoyment for years to come. Risottos are also a great way for kids, once they get older, to have fun and help in the kitchen by assuming stirring duties.

▶ In a medium saucepan, bring chicken broth to a low simmer.

▶ Melt the butter in a separate four-quart saucepan over medium heat.

▶ Add the onion and a pinch of salt to the butter and cook, stirring occasionally, until the onion is soft.

▶ Add the rice and stir until coated with butter and onion mixture. Cook for five minutes.

▶ Add the wine and stir until it is incorporated and cook for a couple of minutes to help alcohol cook off.

Add three cups of the broth and stir until the liquid is absorbed, about ten minutes. Repeat, using one cup of broth and cook stirring frequently. Repeat until rice is cooked but still has a little bite in its center.

Stir in cheese, chicken, artichoke, and baby spinach. Add salt and black pepper to taste.

Serve immediately in shallow bowls.

LENTIL SOUP

SERVES: two to four

RATING: Neanderthal

ESTIMATED PREP AND COOKING TIME: forty-five minutes

TOOLS: knife, spoon

NEED FIRE? yes, on a stovetop

GATHER:

1 tbsp	olive oil
1	large onion, finely chopped
2	medium carrots, chopped
2 ribs	celery, chopped
3 cloves	garlic, minced
1 (14 ½ oz) can	diced tomatoes
1	bay leaf
1 tsp	fresh thyme, minced
1 cup	lentils, rinsed
6 cups	low-sodium chicken broth
1	lemon, juice of
½ cup	fresh parsley, finely chopped
3	scallions, chopped

From prehistoric times until now, soup has been the ultimate comfort food. It's easy to make, a great use for—and source of—leftovers, and with the right ingredients, it can be very healthy. Our prowess as soupmakers has grown over millennia in direct proportion to our skill with tools, to the point where here in the twenty-first century, we have gotten pretty good at it.

Technology is your friend, caveman, so go out and buy yourself an immersion blender, which allows you to either partially or fully puree soup without having to transfer the precooked broth from its original bowl to a blender or food processor.

Lentils are loaded with fiber and iron, so they rank as a nutritional powerhouse for the pregnant woman.

▶ Heat olive oil in stockpot on medium heat and add onion, carrot, and celery, stirring occasionally until the vegetables begin to soften, about four to five minutes.

▶ Add the garlic and cook for another minute.

▶ Add the tomato, bay leaf, and thyme and let cook for two minutes, stirring occasionally.

▶ Add the lentils and salt and pepper to taste. Cook for five minutes.

▶ Add the chicken stock and bring to a boil.

▶ Reduce the heat and simmer until the lentils are tender.

▶ Add the lemon juice, parsley, and scallions.

▶ Serve immediately.

ASPARAGUS SOUP

SERVES: two to four

RATING: Knuckledragger

ESTIMATED PREP AND COOKING TIME: thirty-five minutes

TOOLS: large saucepan, knife, spoon

NEED FIRE? yes, on a stovetop

HUNT:

1 lb	jumbo shrimp, peeled and deveined

GATHER:

¼ cup (½ stick)	unsalted butter
1	large onion, chopped
4 cups	low-sodium chicken broth
1 lb	fresh asparagus
⅓ cup	buttermilk
	salt and pepper to taste

The ingredients in this simple soup are powerhouses in terms of their nutritional value to the expectant mom and the caveling inside her. This particular recipe is made to be flexible, allowing you to substitute almost any vegetable with great results, including carrots, mushrooms, broccoli, celery, cauliflower, beets, and roasted eggplant, to name a few. Pureed vegetable soups are wonderful to serve hot or chilled.

- In a large saucepan, melt butter over medium heat. Add onion and cook until translucent, stirring occasionally. Add chicken broth and bring to a boil.

- Trim tips from asparagus and reserve. Snap off and discard the woody ends (one inch or so). Cut remaining spears into half-inch pieces and drop into boiling broth mixture.

- Cover and reduce heat, simmering for ten to twelve minutes.

- Puree with an immersion blender. Add tips and cook another three minutes.

- Add salt and freshly ground pepper to taste.

TIP: There are many ways to thicken soup. A roux made with equal parts flour and butter is wonderful as a thickener but high in fat. For this recipe, you can use a roux (either at the beginning or the end of the cooking process) or a cornstarch slurry, which is added after the soup is prepared. Just combine equal parts cornstarch and water (start with a couple tablespoons of each) and stir together until starch is dissolved. Whisk slurry into soup until you have achieved your desired thickness and consistency.

PONDER THIS

EVEN YOU CAN DO ROUX

If you thought roux (pronounced "roo") was merely one of Winnie the Pooh's sidekicks, we're here to show you what the Cajuns mean by the word. Often in Cajun meals such as gumbo, a roux is a cooked amalgamation of fat and flour (equal parts by weight) used as a thickening agent in soups and sauces. It can be white, blond, or brown, depending on how long you cook the paste. Cooking the flour in fat coats the starch granules, which prevents lumps from forming. To make a roux, melt butter in a saucepan, then stir in the flour. Keep stirring the mixture over medium heat until the desired color has been reached. A light caramel color is typically a good objective.

SALAD DAYS

Hey, I said I wanted some ketchup! I'm having a salad here!

—HOMER J. SIMPSON, *THE SIMPSONS*

For some reason, our society associates meat-eating with manhood. So when a guy says all he wants is a salad, he may be wrongly subjected to harassment from his brethren. But men who regularly eat salads may have the last laugh, because eating a healthier diet that includes vegetables can translate into a longer lifespan.

The macho man's dismissive attitude toward all things green ignores the nature of our omnivorous Cro-Magnon ancestry. Sure, they would slaughter a bison, butcher the beast, and cook it over fire, then pay the gods homage once the meal was over. But what did they eat with their kill? The accompaniment to the meal consisted of anything clan gatherers could forage: plants, nuts, and fruits. That's right manly-man, Cro-Magnons loved eating salads, and we think the cultivated modern caveman will, too. Salads are seen most frequently as side dishes, but they also make perfect backdrops upon which to feature succulent meats, seafood, or tofu. Furthermore, there is no meal that meets the requirements of the pregnant woman as well as a big salad containing a good variety of vegetables and topped with a healthy dose of protein. Whether as a side dish or a main meal, salads are an excellent choice and are sure to be a consistent crowd-pleaser for your little but growing clan.

Today, salads are easier than ever to prepare because we're blessed in this day and age to have access to virtually every vegetable imaginable at the local grocery store or specialty market. Add to the plethora of veggie options the advent of convenient, pre-packaged lettuces and there is no reason you can't assemble a great salad any night.

Whether you like romaine or spring mix, ready-to-use prewashed lettuce choices abound at the local grocery. Though you pay a higher price for the added convenience, prepackaged lettuce is probably worth it.

The combinations of salad ingredients are endless, so experimentation is highly recommended. There are a couple of good recipes provided here, but be encouraged to pick any ingredients to invent your own healthy and delicious meal. Choose an ingredient or two from each column of the "salad grid" and you will be rewarded with praise and accolades. It will be a true awakening (read: a cold day in hell) when your friends come over to watch the big game and you break out a super bowl of salad. Well, come to think of it, you also might want to supply some chicken wings, nachos, and poppers to satisfy the roomful of hungry knuckledraggers.

ABOUT SALAD DRESSINGS

The most common dressing for salad is the vinaigrette. Vinaigrettes are composed of oil, acid (not the kind found in batteries or at jam-band concerts but that contained in

THE SALAD GRID

SALAD GREENS	VEGETABLES (RAW)	VEGETABLES, (COOKED, PICKLED OR CANNED)	PROTEIN FOODS	FRUITS AND NUTS 1	FRUITS AND NUTS 2
Arugula	Avocado	Artichoke hearts	Bacon	Almonds	Mango
Boston	Bean Sprouts	Asparagus	Cheddar	Apples	Melon
Chicory	Broccoli	Beans	Chicken	Apricots	Papaya
Dandelion greens	Cabbage	Beets	Feta (pasteurized)	Bananas	Peaches
Endive	Carrots	Carrots	Fontina	Berries	Pears
Escarole	Cauliflower	Cauliflower	Hard-boiled egg	Cherries	Persimmon
Frisse	Celery	Corn	Mozzarella	Coconut	Pignoli (pine nuts)
Iceberg	Cucumbers	Hearts of palm	Parmesan	Currants	Pineapple
Radicchio	Mushrooms	Leeks	Pork tenderloin	Dates, figs	Plums
Romaine	Onions and scallions	Olives	Roast beef	Grapefruit	Prunes
Spinach	Peppers, bell	Peas	Cooked salmon	Grapes	Pome-granates
Watercress	Radishes	Peppers, roasted	Cooked trout	Kiwi	Raisins
Fresh herbs	Tomatoes	Potatoes	Tuna	Macadamia Nuts	Walnuts

vinegar and citrus juice), and seasonings. The ratio of oil to acid depends on personal preference and the type of acid being used. The classic ratio of oil to vinegar in French dressings is three to one. However, vinegar may be twice as acidic as fresh citrus juice, so a lime or lemon vinaigrette may contain a higher ratio of acidic ingredients. Again, there is no "right" ratio, so taste frequently to determine your, or rather, her, favorite dressing.

When making dressing, we prefer to use good quality olive oil (extra virgin variety) instead of salad oil to increase the health benefits for a soon-to-be mom. Olive oil contains fats that are good for storing energy for mom and baby. It tastes better, too.

BASIC VINAIGRETTE

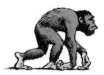

RATING: Knuckledragger

ESTIMATED PREP AND COOKING TIME: less than five minutes

TOOLS: whisk, measuring cup, measuring spoons

NEED FIRE? no

GATHER:

¼ cup	red wine vinegar (balsamic, apple cider, white wine, and sherry vinegars if preferred)
¾ cup	extra virgin olive oil
½ tsp	salt
	freshly ground pepper to taste

▶ Combine vinegar salt and pepper.

▶ Pouring slowly, whisk the olive oil into the vinegar mixture. Adjust seasoning and acidity to taste.

An alternative to the classic "bowl and whisk" method of vinaigrette preparation is to combine all ingredients in a cleaned jar (a mustard jar, for example) and shake vigorously. Yes, caveman, you need the lid tightly on the jar. We recommend this method because it reduces mess and provides an instant storage container.

VARIATIONS ON VINAIGRETTE

MUSTARD VINAIGRETTE: Add one teaspoon of mustard to basic vinaigrette.

HERBED VINAIGRETTE: Add to basic or mustard variation a half-teaspoon fresh herbs.

ITALIAN DRESSING: Add minced garlic, oregano, and parsley.

AVOCADO DRESSING: Puree meat from one avocado into basic recipe. Add lime, salt, and freshly ground pepper to taste.

LIME OR LEMON VINAIGRETTE: Substitute citrus juice with some zest in addition to or in place of vinegar.

GRILLED PORK TENDERLOIN SALAD WITH FRESH MANGO SALSA AND LIME VINAIGRETTE

SERVES: four to six

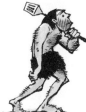

RATING: *Homo habilis*

ESTIMATED PREP AND COOKING TIME: one hour

TOOLS: knife, tongs

NEED FIRE? yes, grill

HUNT:

2 (approx 2 lbs) pork tenderloins

GATHER:

southwest rub (see flank steak recipe, p. 143)

1 mango, diced

1 red bell pepper, chopped

1 jalapeño, diced

1 small onion, diced

¼ cup cilantro, chopped

2 limes, juice from

salt and pepper to taste

As the name indicates, pork tenderloin is a lean, tender cut that is perfectly suited for grilling. It's not the most flavorful cut of pork, but it absorbs spice rubs and marinades very well. Because the cut is so lean, there is little marbling of fat, which means the meat can get very dry if overcooked. So keep the instant-read thermometer handy and remove the tenderloin from the grill when it reads 155° to 160°. Remember, the cooking process continues after removal from the grill, so the temperature will be well into the recommended "safe zone." The mango salsa and lime vinaigrette add moisture to the dish if the medium-well temperature dries the pork slightly.

Pork tenderloin is usually packaged ready to cook. The only prep is removing the elasticlike band at the end of the loin called the silver skin. To remove it, just slip a knife underneath and slide the knife away from you, shallowly slicing it away.

For lime vinaigrette, follow the recipe for classic vinaigrette, but substitute fresh-squeezed lime juice and some lime zest for the vinegar.

FOR THE PORK

- First remove the silver skin.

- Liberally coat tenderloin with Southwest rub.

- Sear pork on medium-hot grill on all sides.

- Move to a cooler part of the grill and cook until internal temperature reaches 160°.

- Remove from grill and let rest five to ten minutes.

- Cut tenderloin into three-quarter-inch slices.

FRESH MANGO SALSA

Mangoes are more widely available today than ever before. Some cooks avoid them because they think mangoes, with their inedible skin and large pit, are too hard too handle. That's not true, even for the digitally clumsy caveman. Handling mangoes actually is pretty straightforward.

- First cut off both ends of the mango so it can be worked with on a flat surface.

- Next, slice off strips of skin from top to bottom. Rotate the mango and slice the skin off until you are left with the orange flesh surrounding the large pit.

- Finally, slice the fruit off, getting as close to the pit as possible.

- Now you can dice the fruit for the salsa.

- Combine mango, bell pepper, jalapeño, onion, cilantro, lime juice, and salt and pepper to taste. Refrigerate.

To assemble salad, lightly toss your favorite lettuce(s) with lime vinaigrette. Arrange pork over lettuce and top with mango salsa.

MARINATED CUCUMBER AND TOMATO SALAD

SERVES: two to four

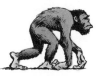

RATING: Knuckledragger

ESTIMATED PREP AND COOKING TIME:
ten minutes

TOOLS: knife, shallow serving dish, bowl

NEED FIRE? no

GATHER:

2	large tomatoes, sliced
1	medium cucumber, sliced
1 tbsp	red wine vinegar
2 tsp	extra virgin olive oil
1	clove garlic, minced
1	lemon, juice of
½	medium red onion, chopped
2 tbsp	fresh basil, minced
	salt and pepper to taste

This simple salad is recommended for summer. Its success hinges on the quality of the vegetables available at your local gathering ground. A farmers' market could be your prime foraging destination.

- Arrange the tomato and cucumbers in a shallow serving dish.

- In a small bowl, combine vinegar, oil, lemon juice, onion, and garlic.

- Pour over cucumber and tomato.

- Add basil, salt, and pepper.

HITTING THE SAUCE

Mankind has a knack for making the most of limited resources. That was the case during the last Ice Age, when our Cro-Magnon ancestors, lacking a proper freezer, used permafrost to store meat after the kill. But after a couple weeks, what happened when whatever meat still left in the makeshift cooler started to turn?

One day, in what was either pure happenstance or brilliant deductive reasoning, a clan elder dropped a piece of overly aged meat into his mead, and all of a sudden, the catch-of-the-day two weeks ago tasted pretty good again. Thus was born the world's first sauce.

The practice of utilizing sauce to disguise bland or tainted meat remained prevalent throughout the centuries. In the first century AD, for example, the great Roman cook and writer Apicius penned *De Re Coquinaria* (On Cookery) and showered his highest praise for one of his best sauces when he triumphantly exclaimed, "No one at the table will know what he's eating."

The culinary caveman should never try to mask his creations, only augment them with more moisture and flavor, while enhancing plate presentation with added colors. A sauce can be as simple as a squeeze of lemon or so complex it requires all day to prepare. We recommend keeping it simple and healthy.

Over many millennia of food preparation, cavemen from disparate cultures across the globe have developed and perfected sauce-making techniques using their own uniquely primitive tools, many of which still have practical applications today, including:

▶ **MORTAR AND PESTLE:** Here's the ideal implement for the budding caveman cook whose knife skills are still developing. A mortar is a bowl, usually made of stone, ceramic or marble. The pestle is a miniature club or bat used to grind and/or pulverize the contents of the mortar—grains, corn, herbs, and the like. Dating back some 6,000 years, the mortar and pestle also have traditionally been used to make medicines.

▶ **MOLCAJETA:** The Central American version of the mortar and pestle, made from stone, often shaped like a pig.

▶ **SURIBACHI AND SURIKOGI:** In the Japanese version of the SATs, suribachi is to mortar as surikogi is to pestle. While these tools are associated with Japanese cuisine, they originated in southern China in the eleventh century. Originally used for grinding herbs for medicine, they are now staples in most Japanese homes.

Whatever the caveman's culinary inclinations, a well-made sauce can be the missing ingredient that transforms a mediocre meal into a great one, a too-dry and flavorless piece of meat into an eminently edible one.

PESTO

SERVES: two to four

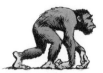

RATING: Knuckledragger

ESTIMATED PREP AND COOKING TIME:
fifteen minutes

TOOLS: mortar and pestle, knife

NEED FIRE? no

GATHER:

3–4	garlic cloves
1 tsp	kosher or coarse sea salt,
1 cup	fresh basil leaves, loosely packed
¼ cup	pine nuts (pignoli)
	Parmigiano Reggiano (high-quality Parmesan cheese), grated, to taste
	extra virgin olive oil, drizzle into the mortar (bowl) until it has the consistency of a smooth paste

Pesto is one of the oldest and most revered sauces on the planet. It's name is derived from its method of preparation: *pestare*, in Italian, means "to pound" or "to grind," as in grinding the ingredients with mortar and pestle. Native to the Liguria region of Italy, pesto, like most Italian cuisine, is best prepared simply and with the highest quality ingredients. A simple pesto is sublime if made with the freshest herbs, the best cheese, and a high-quality olive oil. It can be average, at best, if you skimp on the quality of the ingredients.

A food processor may be used for preparing pestos, but true aficionados know that herbs release more flavor when the leaves are smeared—as with a mortar and pestle—as opposed to cut by a blade. Many also believe the heat created by the whirling electric blade negatively affects the oil in the dish. We feel the rudimentary grinding of ingredients will bring us closer to our ancestry and ultimately provide greater satisfaction in both preparation and consumption.

Pesto has traditionally been served on pasta, which provides a stellar accompaniment to this perfectly simple yet elegant sauce. We also think it a perfect complement to grilled fish and meats, as well as a nice condiment or dressing on sandwiches and salads.

- Put garlic and salt in the mortar and mash into a paste with pestle.

- Add half the basil, half the pine nuts, and some olive oil, and grind and turn the pestle into the ingredients as if you were stirring paint in a gallon can (a skill with which you will soon become accustomed).

- Add the remaining basil, pine nuts, and Parmesan cheese, then grind with more olive oil until you have a smooth sauce.

- Add freshly ground pepper to taste.

The salt you used as an abrasive and the salty Parmesan should provide plenty of salt for the pesto.

HINT: Branch out from the traditional basil pesto by substituting fresh cilantro for the basil. Add some coconut milk (plus chiles if your lady likes it spicy or if she's applying heat to hurry the baby out of the womb) and you have a wonderful Thai sauce in the making.

GRILLED SALSA

SERVES: four to six

RATING: Neanderthal

ESTIMATED PREP AND COOKING TIME: thirty minutes

TOOLS: knife, molcajeta or food processor

NEED FIRE? yes, grill

GATHER:

4	medium plum tomatoes, halved
1	large onion, peeled and halved
1	jalapeño pepper, halved
1	habanero pepper, whole
2	limes, halved, skin side down
¼ cup	cilantro (to taste)
	salt and pepper to taste

While Italians gave us pesto with their mortars and pestles, other cultures work their special ingredients into sauces in the same manner. For thousands of years, people in Central and South America have been grinding food in their pig-shaped molcajeta bowls. Tourists from all over the world take home beautiful, handmade molcajetas, unaware that these pieces actually have a function other than holding nuts. So if you happen to have a stone pig with a hollowed back in your closet, retrieve it for this recipe. Otherwise, a food processor will work fine in its place.

Grilled salsa is a crowd-pleaser. Not only is grilling the easiest, cleanest, and most visually appealing way to make salsa, it is also the best tasting, to the point where you may never crave the store-bought version again. Check with *mamasita* before adding the chili peppers. She may be in a milder mood. The variations and possibilities with grilled salsas are endless, so explore.

- Arrange tomatoes, onion, jalapeño, habanero, and limes on the grill over high heat.

- Remove ingredients and place in a molcajeta or food processor.

- Squeeze lime juice and add it along with salt and pepper.

- Grind or blend.

PONDER THIS

GREAT BALLS OF FIRE!

Exercise caution when handling hot peppers such as habeñeros and jalapeños. They contain juices and oils that can get on your hands when you cut them or handle them after being cut. If you forget to painstakingly wash, rinse, and dry your hands after cutting and handling hot peppers, you are liable to transfer some of the heat to whatever you touch next. If that's your genitals or eyes, you may be in for some long moments of excruciating discomfort. This is a mistake that many a caveman has made…once.

MOCKTAILS: PART PLACEBO, PART NUTRITIONAL VESSEL

Your woman should be drinking plenty of water during pregnancy because dehydration could lead to terrible constipation or even preterm labor. She probably already knows to drink more when it's very hot outside, when traveling on a plane, and during and after exercising.

Her frequent trips to the bathroom suggest she is well hydrated. That may not always be the case, however, since having a baby in the belly exerts added pressure on her bladder. So while she may have worn a path in the carpet from the bedroom to the bathroom, she still needs to drink her fluids regularly.

She may, however, be eyeing the glass of water you are thrusting at her like Cool Hand Luke looking at his fiftieth egg. Sometimes she needs a healthful beverage other than colorless, odorless H_2O. No pregnant (or non-pregnant) woman would turn down a refreshing, nutritious, colorful, and delicious mocktail to supplement her water intake. She also might appreciate her man supporting her abstinence from alcohol

by making an effort to reproduce some of her favorite drinks, like the ones she had the night of conception (you didn't think you were that good looking, did you?). So break out the blender and have fun with the mocktail.

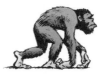

RATING: Knuckledragger

ESTIMATED PREP AND COOKING TIME: five minutes

TOOLS: blender, juice extractor, martini shaker, cool drinking glasses, cocktail/mocktail umbrellas, cool sunglasses

NEED FIRE? no

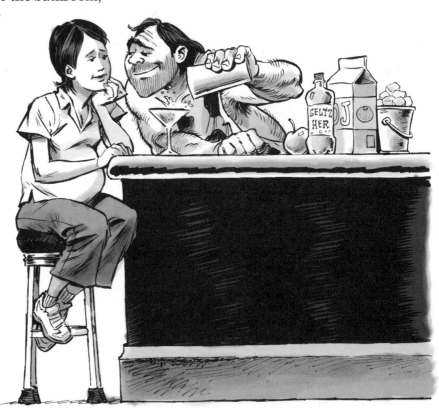

LARGE MARGE-ARITA

SERVES: one

GATHER:

3 oz	fresh-squeezed orange juice
2 oz	fresh-squeezed lime juice
1 oz	sour mix
	coarse salt
	lime wedge
	ice

What makes this take on the classic margarita so good is fresh juices. There is no adequate substitute for freshly squeezed fruit juice.

▶ Blend with ice until smooth.

▶ Serve in a salt-rimmed margarita glass.

▶ Garnish with fresh lime wedge.

PONDER THIS

OCTANE INFUSION

The clever caveman will be sure to double the mocktail recipe and then set aside some of the concoction for his own consumption, knowing full well he can add a little rum, vodka, or tequila and change the "mock" to "cock." In making the effort to become a stellar cook and meal creator, he has earned the right to do so.

MANHATTAN

SERVES: one

GATHER:

2 oz	cranberry juice
2 oz	fresh-squeezed orange juice
1 dash	grenadine
	ice
	lemon
	ice

▶ Mix well, over ice, in a martini shaker.

▶ Serve in a chilled martini glass.

▶ Garnish with lemon twist.

PINÃ COLADA

SERVES: one

GATHER:

3 oz	pineapple juice
2 oz	cream of coconut (store bought, comes in a can)
	whipped cream
	ice
	pineapple, fresh
	cherry

▶ Blend juice with ice in a blender until smooth.

▶ Serve in a hurricane glass and garnish with pineapple wedge, whipped cream, and cherry.

CRANBERRY COOLER

SERVES: one

GATHER:

3 oz	cranberry juice
3 oz	club soda or seltzer
	ice
	lime wedge

➤ Mix well and pour in a tall glass filled with ice.

➤ Serve with a wedge of lime.

GRONK'S FAVORITE SMOOTHIE

SERVES: one

GATHER:

1	banana
3	medium strawberries
8 oz	yogurt, any flavor
6 oz	apple juice
2–3 cubes	ice, just enough to make the drink cold

A superior smoothie is easier to find at home than at the local smoothie stand. The average smoothie on the street typically consists of cloyingly sweet syrup, ice, and frozen yogurt. The key to making a great smoothie at home is simplicity. Use quality fresh fruit, pure juice, yogurt, and just enough ice to make the drink cold. This smoothie, with all its vitamin C, potassium, and calcium, packs a nutritional wallop for mom and baby. Smoothies provide a golden opportunity to try different ingredient combinations, so let 'er rip.

➤ Combine all ingredients in a blender and blend until smooth.

...AND ONE FOR THE CAVEMAN

WARNING: THIS TEA IS FULL PROOF! (NOT FOR MOMMIES-TO-BE)

GOOD TIMES: FAVORITE STRESS-RELIEVING TEA

SERVES: one

GATHER:

1 oz	vodka
1 oz	gin
1 oz	light rum
1 oz	tequila
1 oz	sour mix
	cola, to turn drink color of tea

Except for the vodka, gin, and tequila, it's exactly like real tea! After a tough day, hide your car keys and try this refreshing take on traditional iced tea, the Long Island iced tea. No need for top-shelf ingredients; well caliber works fine. The result is a beverage that tastes much like traditional iced tea. No refills on this one, however.

➤ Shake all ingredients except cola and pour over ice in a tall glass.

➤ Add cola and garnish with lemon wedge.

FOOD FOR THOUGHT...

Back in prehistoric times, the Cro-Magnon hunter who risked life and limb to bring big game such as reindeer and bison back to the stone domicile earned special stature in the clan. Similarly, the guy who masters the preceding recipes and becomes self-sufficient in the kitchen stands to be honored as his family's Grand Provider and an übercaveman.

Now, having passed your crash course in kitchen proficiency, the only thing standing between you and your ascendance to true cultivated cavedad status is the birth of your child. That bun in the oven is nearly done cooking. Prepare yourself, for this final test likely will be the toughest. Both you and your woman will need to eat heartily and healthily in preparation for the childbirth challenge ahead.

CHAPTER 7

THE NEONATAL NEANDERTHAL

Well, there's a child on the way
It could be any day
But how this life will change him
That we don't know
Well, there's a child on the way
Gonna look just like him
One day, he's gonna say,
"Ain't you my dad?"

—WILCO, "DREAMER IN MY DREAMS"

ALMOST FORTY WEEKS have passed since you unscrewed a bottle of vino, lit some musk-scented incense, led your woman to the *faux* bearskin rug, and a while later, sent your intrepid sperm to meet their destiny. Some nine months after one of your little swimmers hit its mark and joined with the awaiting egg to make an embryo, a faint light now flickers at the end of the pregnancy tunnel.

But first the small matter of bringing a baby into the world. It has been a rigorous but rewarding three trimesters for you and your partner. With the cultivated caveman Gronk as your guide, you have managed to evolve into a competent, cultivated cave-dad-to-be in your own right, a Renaissance

GROW WITH GRONK

What the caveman stands to gain from reading Chapter 7:

▶ **EXPLANATIONS** of some of the key issues confronting him during labor and childbirth

▶ **A KNOWLEDGE** of conventional and unconventional birthing options

▶ **THE ABILITY** to distinguish between indications of true and false labor

▶ **A FIRM UNDERSTANDING** of his role during labor and delivery

▶ **AN IN-DEPTH KNOWLEDGE** of the entire labor and delivery process, including potential complications and procedures along the way

▶ **THE KNOW-HOW** to help his woman during labor's difficult moments

▶ **INSIGHT** into the key role nurses play in labor, delivery, and postpartum

▶ **A WORKING KNOWLEDGE** of the drugs and instruments that could be deployed during labor and delivery

▶ **A CLEAR IDEA** of what happens after his child is delivered

▶ **A SENSE** of what lies ahead for him as a parent

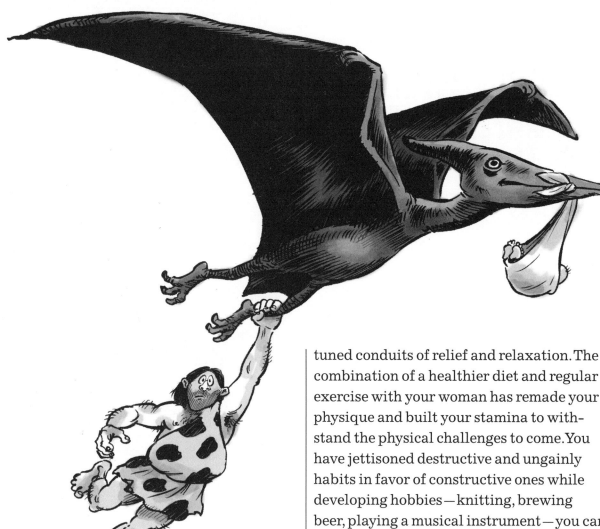

rockhead who is as ready as he will ever be to embrace the responsibilities of parenthood. Following Gronk's example, you have turned yourself into a respectable and prolific meal-making machine. You have learned a series of prenatal massage maneuvers that have transformed your hands from clumsy, callused appendages into skilled, finely tuned conduits of relief and relaxation. The combination of a healthier diet and regular exercise with your woman has remade your physique and built your stamina to withstand the physical challenges to come. You have jettisoned destructive and ungainly habits in favor of constructive ones while developing hobbies—knitting, brewing beer, playing a musical instrument—you can enjoy for a lifetime.

Meanwhile, you and your woman have spent long hours preparing your home and its contents for the pterodactyl's arrival. You have toured the birthing facility, met members of the baby-catching squad, packed your hospital bag, arranged a postpartum baby visitation schedule for family and friends, assembled a crib and various other pieces of gear and furniture, and installed a car seat.

PONDER THIS

CAVEMAN WITH A PLAN

The wrenching twists and turns of the labor and birthing experience can bring even the strongest caveman to his knees. Assuming that at various points during the process you will feel physically exhausted, emotionally overtaxed, and thus unable to think clearly, and assuming your woman will be focused more on the momentous task at hand, what happens when there are important decisions to be made or key steps to be taken, but neither of you is in a position to decisively deal with the situation?

It is in these situations that having a birthing plan in place proves to be a huge help. A birthing plan is a relatively short document the two of you draft ahead of time in which you express your preferences and vision for the labor and birthing process. By making the effort to draft such a plan, you and other members of the birthing squad have a clear written statement of your intentions when, for whatever reason, in the heat of the moment, you can't find the words to lucidly state those intentions yourself. With so much information to process, a potentially overmatched caveman now has a tip sheet to which he and others can refer when his mind draws a blank.

A birthing plan should be flexible to accommodate the changeable conditions common to labor and childbirth. In it you will address such things as:

▶ Who you want in the delivery room with you

▶ Your preferences with regard to variables like use of fetal heart-monitoring instruments, episiotomy, epidural injection, and other pain medications. You and your woman may feel strongly on such issues as natural (drug-free) childbirth and episiotomy. Here is where you state those inclinations.

▶ How you want your care providers to handle complications should they arise, being aware that issues of legal liability could come into play.

▶ Who you want as part of the birthing squad (perhaps a doula or midwife)

▶ The methods and positions you plan to use during labor to relieve pain and discomfort (massage, bath, breathing exercises, hypnosis, etc.)

▶ Your woman's preferred birthing position

▶ The sort of environment you want for the birth (music or quiet, strong lighting or soft)

▶ If it's a boy, whether you will have him circumcised

Once you have a plan in place, type it up, print out a bunch of copies, and pack them in your hospital bag so you can distribute them once you arrive there for the big event.

Through it all, though both of you have been exceedingly busy and often tired (especially the expectant mom), you have not only managed to find time for sleep, but also maintained your sanity by making a point of doing the things you like to do as a couple and as individuals.

This is an awful lot for a guy to accomplish in a matter of forty weeks. You are a caveman, not a superman, and Gronk is a tough act to follow. So don't put too much pressure on you and your woman to do absolutely everything or too much at once as the due date approaches. With all he accomplished when his woman was with child, Gronk represents the gold standard for expectant fathers. All we ask is that you, as a disciple of Gronk, do your best to follow in his footsteps.

Amid all the prenatal activity—and with the help of the birthing class you and your woman may have attended, plus discussions with friends and family—the two of you have been gradually growing accustomed to the idea of being parents, to the point where you are confident and ready to tackle one of the biggest challenges of your lives.

What's more, you, the newly cultivated caveman, have more than pulled your weight during these nine months, earning accolades from your woman and everyone else who has witnessed your impressive embrace of expectant parenthood and the incredible evolutionary steps you have taken in a relatively short span of time. It is with a justified sense of pride that you and your woman pronounce yourselves ready for the package to drop.

With your woman's due date now close at hand, you have made every effort to tie up loose ends:

- ▸ **PACKED** a bag to bring to the birthing facility (see p. 175 for suggestions on exactly what to pack)

- ▸ **GATHERED** your massage tools and reconditioned your hands so they're ready for action, especially if labor runs long

- ▸ **COMPILED** your In Utero, in Stereo mix (see p. 39) along with other music selections for the maternity-ward jukebox, your woman having nixed your suggestion that you bring your guitar and supply the music yourself

- ▸ **STOCKED** the fridge and freezer with meals you prepared so they're ready to cook once you arrive home with the baby

- ▸ **PREPARED** some portable snacks to bring to the hospital or birthing facility so you won't have to rely on cafeteria gruel or vending machines as your sole source of nourishment

- ▸ **FINALIZED** plans for someone to care for your pet(s) while you and your woman are busy bringing a child into the world

- ▸ **JOINED** your woman for one last visit to your new favorite place, the day spa

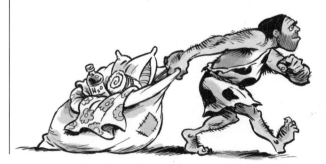

MATERNITY WARD CAMPING KIT

Chances are your woman, newborn, and you will be in the hospital (if that's your chosen birthing venue) for at least a couple days—and perhaps longer. What to pack in your birthing bag of tricks? Here are a few suggestions:

LIGHT SNACKS (nice alternative to cafeteria gruel)

SEVERAL CHANGES OF CLOTHES (comfort-oriented)

DEODORANT, TOOTHBRUSH, TOOTHPASTE, OTHER TOILETRIES

CLOTHING FOR THE BABY (seasonally appropriate)

DIAPERS

READING MATERIAL

MUSIC (and a means to play it if labor/delivery room is lacking)

WATER BOTTLES/BOTTLED WATER

HEADLAMP (for late-night reading if first-stage labor is dragging)

BLACKOUT EYEWEAR

CELL PHONE AND CHARGER

AIR MATTRESS

A GIFT TO GIVE TO YOUR WIFE (jewelry with precious stone is a nice touch)

YOUR OWN PILLOW AND SECURITY BLANKET

CAMERA (film, batteries, charger, memory card)

NURSING BRAS (for her, but may double as blackout eyewear for you)

GOOD BOTTLE OF WINE/CHAMPAGNE (if your woman is up to celebrating in that style)

CIGARS (to give away or to enjoy with friends/family in a designated smoking area)

Now begins the waiting game. And the wait for labor to begin can be agonizing, particularly if the due date has arrived or passed and family members have already descended on your home, expecting the baby to have appeared by now. There may be false starts, with periodic "practice" contractions (Braxton-Hicks contractions) followed by long periods with no clearly evident labor indications whatsoever. These fits and starts, called false labor, can be frustrating and nerve-racking for the expectant couple.

As Dr. Brian notes in the "Cava Sutra" section of Chapter 5, there are ways to take matters in your own hands in an effort to expedite the labor process. If you, like many expectant fathers during the final weeks of pregnancy, have been deprived of any-

DR. BRIAN

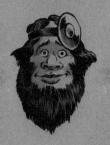

WHEN THE LEVEE BREAKS

*Cryin' won't help you, prayin' won't do you
  no good
Now, cryin' won't help you, prayin' won't do
  you no good
When the levee breaks, mama, you got to move*
  —LED ZEPPELIN,
    "WHEN THE LEVEE BREAKS"

It can be difficult for a caveman to comprehend how a baby survives roughly forty weeks inside the womb of a woman, especially one who is particularly active. When she's walking, working out, engaging in hanky-panky, or going about her daily activities, the safety-minded father-to-be wonders how all this action is affecting the poor fetus. Rest assured, your baby is well protected inside your woman's uterus thanks to the amniotic sac, a thin membrane filled with fluid (and the placenta). It serves as a fetal shock absorber, surrounding the little one with a frequently replenished supply of liquid.

The amniotic fluid makes the baby buoyant inside the bag of waters, providing the caveling with a smooth ride inside the womb even when the going outside gets rough. When a woman's water breaks, labor usually is right around the corner, if it hasn't started already. If contractions don't begin within a specified time after her water breaks, the healthcare team may deem it time for labor to be induced, since the youngster has lost the built-in protection afforded by the fluid.

Should you be ready with galoshes, bucket, and mop for this event? Not necessarily. When your woman reaches term, her amniotic sac may hold as much as a quart of fluid. But fluid can escape the punctured amniotic sac in a trickle or a torrent. So the cue for the caveman to break out in his best Robert Plant croon—and to call the doctor or midwife to tell them what happened—won't necessarily be an obvious splash.

thing resembling sexual intercourse, here's an opportune time (in an act of selfishness cloaked in selflessness) to point out that intercourse, coupled with nipple stimulation and capped by orgasms for both of you, is precisely what's needed to supply her body with the hormonal impetus that can put the process in motion.

CAVEMENSCH

Lawsy, we'se got ter have a doctah. Ah don' know nuthin' 'bout birthin' babies.

—PRISSY, GONE WITH THE WIND

Voila! Within a couple of hours of your strategically motivated sexual encounter (one from which you clearly derived more pleasure than she), her water has broken and she has begun feeling the sharp, regular contractions in her abdomen that are the telltale sign of labor's onset. Anxiety dissolves into a more intense rush of reality. Your first instinct may be to panic or to escape to your safe place—the basement, garage, or other cavelike environment.

Your mind races. Your adrenaline surges. Your heart rate escalates. Your palms sweat. And in your brain the thought registers: this is not a drill; it is first-stage labor. The moment to mobilize has arrived. Here's where three trimesters of physical and mental preparations come to bear. With all you have learned, and with support and guidance from prenatal mentor and kindred caveman spirit Gronk, it is time to stand tall (or at least upright), time to make the rest of the male species proud by supporting your woman as best you can during one of the biggest moments of your life together.

Remain calm, caveman. Your woman is counting on you to think clearly and act decisively on her behalf in the hours to come. The final push to reach the end of the pregnancy tunnel, both literally and figuratively, will be hard on your woman, the fetus, and you. It will likely be exhausting.

Thankfully, you're not the one giving birth. But as the pace of labor ebbs and flows, it is not unusual at various points to feel overwhelmed and tired, euphoric and ecstatic, like you are losing focus or control. That's when you need to recall the yeomanlike efforts of your role models from the animal kingdom—remember the male seahorse, jacana bird, giant water bug, Panamanian poison-arrow frog, emperor penguin, and red fox?—and to remind yourself of the many perks you stand to enjoy as a competent father-to-be. Think of all the lifelong skills you have gained, the benefits of which you and your family will hopefully be reaping for decades to come.

With the approach of labor, it's time for the caveman to step into a supporting role. He's there primarily to help his woman and the team of professionals that will be surrounding her during the process in whatever way he can. A supporting role may feel odd to a guy whose instincts and pride delude him into believing he should be leading this operation. In this case, unless the caveman also happens to be a doula, midwife, registered nurse, or medical doctor (like our own Dr. Brian), he is an important player but a supporting player nonetheless.

Bottom line: this situation is largely out of your control. You are part of a team of people who will be working to ensure the outcome of the experience is positive and the baby is healthy. In some ways you, as the pregnant woman's partner, are the most important member of the team because of the special forms of support—massage, whispered words of comfort, reading, managing the birthing suite musical soundtrack—only you can offer the patient.

With that in mind, as an expectant father whose first moments of fatherhood are fast approaching, you will be donning your caddy and coach hats. While all eyes are on your woman, you will be working behind the scenes, a calm, steadying force who is on call to help wherever needed.

Sports terms are appropriate in describing the caveman's role during the experience. Know your limitations as a supporting player. *Do not* be a liability. Eat well and drink water throughout so you won't wilt prematurely under the heat and pressure. Sit down if you feel wobbly or green. Practice visualization techniques in which you envision yourself calmly coaching your laboring woman and, through sheer will, coaxing your son or daughter out of the uterus, down the birthing canal, and into the light at the end of the tunnel.

It can be challenging to stay coherent during a grueling labor. Do what it takes to stay lucid so you can process information and handle key situations and decisions. Be present in the moment. And most importantly, do not lose consciousness. You need to be awake to offer comfort.

The average labor for a primigravida (first-timer) lasts from eight to fourteen hours. However well prepared you believe you are, the intensity of the labor and delivery experience still may catch you off guard at times. Your preparations, as well as your surroundings and environment, have something to do with how that experience unfolds. What's occurring with your baby and woman will dictate the rest.

ALTERNATIVES TO BIRTHING BY THE BOOK

Back when our knuckledragging ancestors roamed the Earth, childbirth could happen just about anyplace—on a bed of leaves in the forest, in the comforting confines of the clan's cave, wherever the contents of the woman's womb dictated.

In some respects (and in your case, many respects), we aren't too far removed from our prehistoric predecessors. Even today people frequently choose to have their babies outside the conventional facilities to which many of us are accustomed, using practices that don't necessarily conform to mainstream birthing approaches. Gronk, for example, was born in a meadow, by a stream, one summer day in the mid-1970s, when a prenatal hiking excursion by his parents, Lucy and Grulk, turned into a lightning-fast natural childbirth experience, with Grulk, a brick mason by trade, putting his hands to a different but no less constructive use.

Typically practiced in more controlled environments, some alternative approaches like hypnosis birthing and water birthing may have their merits. Here's some background on each, if the two of you are considering alternatives to conventional hospital labor and delivery practices.

BIRTH UNDER HYPNOSIS. It turns out birthing doesn't have to be a painful experience after all. At least that's what some advocates of hypnotic birthing techniques claim.

A woman who can put herself in a deep state of relaxation through self-hypnosis, they say, can better control, even eliminate pain during childbirth because she is less tense and more at ease. Who needs doctor-prescribed pain medication when, through self-hypnosis during labor, a woman's body can release enough natural chemicals to help keep pain at bay? A more relaxed mother during labor and birth, hypnotic birth supporters reason, translates directly into a better experience and outcome for both her and the baby, as well as to a newborn who eats and sleeps better.

Usually pregnant women must attend hypnotic birthing classes to learn self-hypnosis and relaxation techniques such as deep breathing. Many supporters claim hypnosis birthing is rooted in the birthing techniques of our ancient ancestors, so this may indeed be the kind of primal experience the couple is seeking.

WATER BIRTH. Eons ago the primordial oceans gave birth to Earth's first organisms. Here in the twenty-first century, some members of the human species that evolved from the primordial soup are returning to the water to give birth to their offspring.

In a water birth, a woman spends part or all of the labor and delivery process partially submerged in warm water, an environment that purportedly is gentler on the baby because it is similar to conditions in the amniotic sac. A water birth can happen at home or in a properly equipped hospital or birthing center, under the supervision of a doctor, midwife, or other expert. Recent studies have shown that relative to other delivery methods, water birth may shorten the first stage of labor, reduce the rate of episiotomy, and make women less apt to use analgesics for pain relief, all without compromising the safety of the mother or the baby.[1]

Some obstetricians assert that birthing in water, with its soothing powers and the buoyancy it provides, reduces stress on both the baby and mother, resulting in fewer fetal complications.

For couples whose baby was conceived in water (bath tub, hot tub, pool, pond, ocean), water birthing is a way to complete the circle. Water birth isn't for everyone, however, so you and your woman should consult her doctor when considering your birthing options. If your baby is in breech position, for example, or if the expectant mom has toxemia or pre-eclampsia, a water birth may be discouraged.

1. THOENI, A., N. ZECH, L. MORODER, F. PLONER. "Review of 1600 water births. Does water birth increase the risk of neonatal infection?" *Journal of Maternal-Fetal and Neonatal Medicine* (May 2005) Taylor & Francis

PREPAREDNESS DRILL: IS YOUR HEAD IN THE GAME?

Mental preparation is key to being a functional labor and delivery partner. It's therefore wise for the uninitiated caveman to take himself through a labor and delivery dry run that will help him resolve some of his concerns before he and his woman even set foot in the birthing facility. Here are a few questions to ponder beforehand to put yourself in a state of mental readiness.

Q. WHAT'S THAT COMPUTER-LOOKING THING IN THE CORNER?

When you enter the delivery room for the first time, you're likely to observe a variety of high-tech machines, one being a computer-like device with a screen, a small printer, and two belts attached. This is an **electronic fetal heart-rate monitor** (EFM), which is used in at least 80 percent of all births in the United States. The belts, which are wrapped around the woman's abdomen, monitor the relationship between contractions and the baby's heart rate to give the caregiver a baseline of activity from the mom and baby. Depending on various risk factors and the medical team's inclinations, some caregivers choose to keep the monitor on throughout labor (continuous EFM), but most will get the baseline readout, then check the heart rate intermittently after that. This allows mom to move about more freely during labor. The screen shows contraction activity and the fetal heart rate simultaneously and continuously, while the printer is like the sports ticker, spitting out a steady stream of documentation.

Q. WHAT ARE THOSE IMPOSING-LOOKING INSTRUMENTS ON THE TRAY OVER THERE?

Only since the last generation have men been allowed into delivery rooms. And for good reason: many of them are prone to fainting at the sight of large needles and invasive instruments. For example, an epidural syringe looks big enough to vaccinate King Kong, and the needle attached to it looks like it belongs atop the Empire State Building. Then there are the tools used in assisted deliveries. To the uninitiated, **forceps** look like sadistic salad tongs; watching them in use can be rather unsettling, though when wielded by a practiced caregiver, they are extremely safe for extracting the baby from the birth canal.

Q. WHO WILL BE IN THE DELIVERY ROOM WITH US?

Besides the two of you and your care providers (nurses, doctors, doula, midwife, etc.), many birthing facilities give couples discretion to allow friends and family in to view the birth. This is a highly personal decision that the two of you should talk about ahead of time. In Gronk's case, his suggestion that his poker buddies be on hand in the delivery room to film the event was dismissed without debate. In your situation, if the two of you opt to invite friends and family to witness the action as VIPs (Viewers of Intense Pain), it's wise to write the roster down as part of your birthing plan and furnish it to members of the labor and delivery team so there will be no debate or confrontations in the heat of labor.

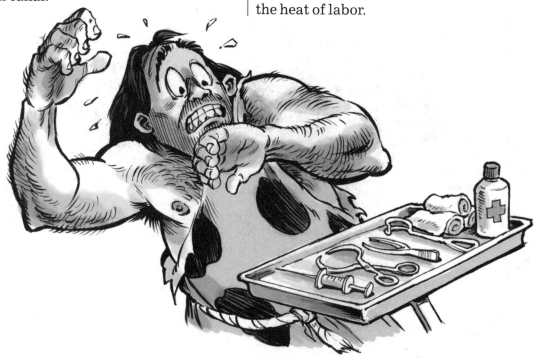

Q. WHAT WILL BE MY CAPACITY FOR GRAPHIC VIEWING?

How close a view you get of the goings-on in your woman's pelvic region depends on how much your woman wants you to see and how much you think you can take. Delivery can put your woman in the most compromising of positions. Fluids will be flowing, muscles will be stretching to or beyond the breaking point, and large needles and other intimidating devices could be used on your woman (see above). These are not sights for the squeamish. If you're curious, you have a stomach for that kind of stuff, and your woman clears you for up-close spectating, go for it. If you think you lack the fortitude or your woman, out of a sense of modesty or privacy, demands you watch from a distance, then adjust your view accordingly.

Q. WHAT'S THE DEAL WITH UMBILICAL CORD BLOOD?

There's a new kind of bank in town, and it's not used for money or sperm but to store umbilical cord blood drawn from newborns. Parents now face a choice about whether to "bank" their little caveling's umbilical cord blood for potential use in treating future illness. Since 1988, cord blood cells have been successfully transplanted in patients with diseases such as leukemia to repopulate depleted bone marrow. And scientific progress points to broader uses for cord blood further into the future, perhaps in your child's lifetime.

Every new parent wishes to give their child every advantage possible in life and cord blood banking has been advertised by commercial blood banks as a necessary purchase for all caring parents. The implication from these companies is that if you choose not to spend the considerable money it takes to bank cord blood, you may be doing your new baby a disservice.

But while cord blood has been used successfully for years in transplants, there is little evidence supporting the notion that you need to bank your child's cord blood for future autologous (defined for the caveman as "from one's own body") procedures. Unlike bone marrow transplants, cord blood is relatively easy to match for successful transplantation, so one's own blood may not be necessary for a successful transplant. A more significant gesture may be to donate cord blood to a larger public registry, where it's more broadly accessible to people who may need it.

What's more, a recent study commissioned by the European Union from the European Group on Ethics (EGE) concludes that "the legitimacy of commercial cord blood banks for autologous use should be questioned as they sell a service which has presently, no real use regarding therapeutic options. Thus, they promise more than they can offer." Other professional organizations that have denounced the privatization of cord blood banking include the American College of Obstetrics (ACOG), the American Academy of Pediatrics (AAP), and the Royal College of

Obstetrics and Gynecology (RCOG). For more information on the subject, start by visiting the National Marrow Donor Program Center for Cord Blood Web site at www.marrow.org/NMDP/center_for_cb.html.

Q. WHAT EXPLAINS MY NEWBORN'S ALIEN APPEARANCE?

Even after a relatively uneventful, complication-free vaginal delivery, the first glimpse of your newborn may be a bit unnerving. You're accustomed to seeing newborns on TV and in the movies that debut as clean, smiling, cooing little cuties. The reality is that your baby will look more like the Hollywood version of an alien: potentially cone-shaped head; deeply wrinkled, blue-tinted skin covered in various liquids; mouth emitting ear-splitting yells. Don't fret, members of the health team will wash the baby, and the baby's head should round out in short time.

NURSES: ANGELS IN WHITE

If there is anyone the caveman would be wise to befriend during his stay at a birthing facility or hospital maternity ward, it is the nurses. They are the ones who will care for your woman, baby, and you virtually from the moment you walk in the door, through labor and delivery, right up until you leave to take Baby Unibrow home. Ask many nurses and they will privately tell you that they, not doctors, are the ones who make the

PONDER THIS

RN RAPPORT

In the nerve-racking and adrenalin-charged moments when you first arrive at the birthing venue, all your focus will be on the well being of your woman. But don't forget your manners, cavelout. It can be difficult to summon the presence of mind to calmly introduce yourself to the nurses who will be attending to your woman in the hours ahead and even harder to remember each of their names. Your efforts to reach out will be appreciated and likely will put you and your brood in the good graces of the nursing staff. And during labor and delivery, you want the nurses on your side.

maternity ward baby-delivery machine tick. And after a few days watching the machine in action, you may tend to agree. Sure, it's the doctor who steals much of the glory by entering during the late moments of labor to deliver the child and announce, "It's a…" That's why they earn the big bucks.

But it's almost always the nurses, not the doctors, who are with you, your partner, and the baby every step of the way during the hospital or birthing facility stay (unless the condition of mother or baby warrant otherwise). During labor and delivery, your woman and the baby inside her will predominately be under the care of labor and delivery nurses—nurses who have been specially trained to help bring your baby into the world. For the bewildered caveman, it's comforting knowing the nurses who surround him are skilled, caring professionals with extensive experience caring for women and babies during labor and delivery. They've been through this process dozens if not hundreds of times, so they are great people to turn to for answers to your questions or just for comfort. Depending on how long labor lasts, you may encounter several shifts of nurses. Among their responsibilities are to monitor the condition of mother and fetus at all times via the various high-tech equipment attached to her and the baby inside her, and to constantly communicate the condition of each to attending doctors, the expectant mom's OB-GYN, and other relevant members of the birthing team. They administer medicine and carry out physicians' orders. They are also there to cater to the expectant mother's needs, ensuring she is as comfortable as possible and progressing through the sometimes lengthy labor process. And they are there to support and encourage the prehistoric procreator to contribute wherever he can during the process, whether it's daubing his woman's forehead with a cool cloth, leading her through breathing exercises, or holding her hand during delivery.

The expectant father should be the least of the nurses' worries. But in instances when the caveman gets a little queasy or appears to be buckling under the weight of the situation, the nurse is there for him as well, ready with smelling salts, a glass of cold water, or a cot to lie on—basically whatever it takes to ensure the focus of the whole operation remains where it should be, on the woman and not her poor, helpless *Homo habilis*.

Once the miracle has occurred and both mother and baby are safe and stabilized, usually an hour or so after delivery, it's typical for labor and delivery nurses to hand responsibilities over to their postpartum nurse colleagues, who are responsible for caring for the newborn and his or her parents until the end of the stay.

LABOR & DELIVERY: IMMEASURABLE PAIN, IMMEASURABLE GAIN

Oh yes, I am wise
But it's wisdom born of pain
Yes, I've paid the price
But look how much I gained
If I have to, I can do anything
I am strong
I am invincible
I am woman

—HELEN REDDY, "I AM WOMAN"

There's no place quite like a hospital maternity ward. While a hushed quiet prevails in most sections of a typical hospital, the labor, delivery, and nursery areas are usually bustling with activity around the clock, seven days a week, 365 days a years, as women labor and give birth, babies take their first breaths, and caveman dads breathe huge sighs of relief.

Besides crying newborns, sighing new fathers, cooing friends and relatives, and blipping computer-monitoring devices, one sound you are apt to hear consistently in the maternity ward is the roar of laboring and birthing women. In the tremendous and miraculous undertaking that is childbirth, you may have the opportunity to hear your woman—and perhaps women in neighboring birthing suites—unleash a range of roars: a determined one, an accusatory one, a surprised one, a guttural one, a proud one, a pained one, an exhausted one, an exhilarated one.

These roars are just a small sample of the wonders revealed to you during labor and childbirth. For the doctors, nurses, and other birthing professionals in your midst, the labor experience—all three stages of it—is familiar territory. The truly grizzled veterans have been through this hundreds, even thousands of times.

The last labor you experienced, on the other hand, was the one in which you made your own mother roar. This time the woman who is ready to give birth and the child who is poised to make his or her first appearance are your own. Needless to say, the wild-eyed look on your face says you are a first-timer.

Your cause isn't helped by the fact that you occasionally let your attention wander during birthing class. You're left with only a vague idea of how to recognize the signs labor has begun and, once it is officially confirmed that your woman is indeed in labor, of how the whole process will unfold. Thank-

fully, you have supplemented your class work by reading this book, for in the pages that follow, the mysteries of labor will be explained in terms a greenhorn like you can understand.

Labor is typically divided into three stages, first, second, and third. There's little telling how long each stage will last, although the first stage typically takes longer than the two others. The lengthy first stage is when your woman must endure the most intense contractions as her cervix and the baby get into position; the second stage is when she actually begins pushing in earnest and delivers the child; the third stage is when she delivers the placenta.

This is a distance race, not a sprint, so pace yourself. If things go perfectly—if the cervix behaves as expected, if mom manages her pain well, if the baby is in a favorable head-down birthing position and has a relatively uneventful trip through the birthing canal—the process may progress and conclude rather expeditiously, in a matter of hours, not days. However, many couples find that with so many variables in play, labor and delivery don't always go as the textbooks say they should.

Labor's first stage is when you will begin conversing with other members of the birthing squad in the language of labor and delivery, showing off all the terms you have recently added to your vocabulary, among them:

DILATION: A measurement of the opening of the cervix, expressed in centimeters

EFFACEMENT: A measurement of the extent to which the cervix has flattened, expressed as a percentage

RIPENING: The softening of the cervix that makes dilation and effacement possible

STATION: The location of the baby's head relative to certain points in the woman's pelvis, measured on a scale of zero to plus five, with the high end of the scale meaning the head is in crowning position at the opening of the vagina

PRESENTATION: The part of the baby presenting itself to exit first—head, bottom, etc.

POSITION: An indication of which way the baby's presenting part (usual the head) is facing

Vocabulary isn't the only skill the caveman has to dust off during this crucial time. He also needs to demonstrate his grasp of basic math and measuring skills because throughout labor, the medical team will be throwing numbers at him, such that he will begin to feel as if he is monitoring the score of a game on the television sports ticker: "She's five centimeters dilated and 70 percent effaced, the baby is at station three. Contractions are measured one minute long and three minutes apart." In this case you and other members of the labor and delivery squad are tracking scores that indicate your woman's progress toward the next stage of labor and your baby's progress toward, down, and ultimately out of the birthing canal.

PONDER THIS

GRONK'S DILATION GAUGE

Hearing that a pregnant woman's cervix is dilated to a certain number of centimeters means little to the metrically challenged caveman. What he needs is a means of pegging the width of his woman's cervical opening—and thus the proximity or progress of labor—to familiar items from his unique universe.

1 CM = M&M candy

2 CM = pistachio nut

3 CM = No. 2 wooly bugger fly

4 CM = diameter of shot glass opening

5 CM = diameter of poker chip

6 CM = three fingers of whiskey

7 CM = buffalo wing

8 CM = diameter, drinking end of pint glass

9 CM = length of longest chest hair

10 CM = diameter of golf cup

DR. BRIAN

5-1-1: THE RULES OF CONTRACTION

Among all the indications that true labor has begun, having consistent contractions is perhaps the strongest. So if you and your woman are wondering if now is the right time to call your doctor, midwife, doula, etc., you need to be aware of the 5-1-1 Rule. It's a general rule of thumb that most medical professionals suggest their pregnant patients follow. You will need a watch, clock, or other time-keeping device (preferably with a second hand) to measure the time from the beginning of one contraction to the beginning of the next, the duration of a single contraction, and the period of time during which those contractions have been occurring. When you find contractions to be happening 5 minutes apart, lasting for 1 minute, and having been occurring consistently for 1 hour, it's time to make the call and get ready for your ride to the birthing facility.

TRUE OR FALSE?

But let's not get too far ahead of ourselves. First the two of you must resolve a major question: are the symptoms your woman is experiencing indicative of true labor or merely the signs of false labor? This may be the toughest true-false question the caveman has ever had to answer.

True labor is confirmed by the emergence of consistent contractions coupled with an internal examination of the cervix. Although you are somewhat familiar with that area of your woman's body and you have a ruler that measures in centimeters, this endeavor is best left to medical experts, not enthusiastic volunteers like yourself. Such examinations reveal the extent to which your woman is effaced and dilated. In the weeks and days leading up to labor, your woman will return from her frequent pelvic exams to report a fresh set of numbers indicating any progress made by her cervix. Eventually, you will hear members of the labor and delivery team report the same types of numbers, so you should be well versed in their meaning. A cervix that has not begun to flatten is 0-percent effaced. A cervix that has completely flattened is considered 100-percent effaced. As the cervix opens it also begins to dilate; dilation is measured on a scale from zero to ten centimeters, so that when she is fully dilated at ten centimeters (about four inches), the cervix has opened to roughly the width of a golf cup.

If the two of you are unsure whether it's true labor or false, even after reading some

THIS IS NOT A DRILL—OR IS IT?

TRUE LABOR	FALSE (PRE/PRACTICE) LABOR
Contractions have become regular, increasing in duration, intensity, frequency	Contractions come inconsistently, with duration and intervals in between varying; not too painful; feel more like Braxton-Hicks contractions
Contractions show pattern of progress, getting closer together	No pattern of progression evident; contractions irregular
Contractions persist through (and even worsen from) woman's activity and her changes of position	Activities such as walking or a change in position reduce or stop contraction activity
Likelihood of bloody show	No bloody show
Likelihood of water breaking	Water has not broken
Woman feels contractions most acutely in higher part of uterus/abdomen	Woman feel contractions most acutely in lower part of uterus/abdomen
Pain from contraction radiates	Pain from contraction is more localized
Progress in effacement, dilation of cervix	Little or no progress in effacement, dilation

of the key distinctions listed above, it is crucial for you to consult your medical care provider. They may want your woman to come in for a precautionary examination. Even if the examination shows that it was just a false start, keep in mind that false labor is a constructive activity because it helps prepare your woman's body for the real thing.

Every labor is different, so while you may find it sporting to try to predict how your woman's cervix measurements will progress during the late stages of pregnancy, it will be next to impossible to do so accurately. Some women are like fine sports cars, with

the ability to quickly accelerate from zero to ten. Others take awhile to get off the starting line, with the cervix effacing and dilating gradually over a period of weeks before labor begins. For some, dilation doesn't begin until the onset of true labor. And in certain situations—such as when a loss of amniotic fluid puts the baby at risk—the doctor may deem it necessary to speed the process by administering a labor-inducing drug such as Pitocin. This is aptly called "inducing" the birth.

Absent the ability to check your woman's cervix and make an indisputable diagnosis that she is in labor, you need to be alert for other telltale signs that distinguish true labor from false. Steady, strengthening contractions are a major indictor that it's the real thing. Factors such as the breaking of the bag of waters (see "Dr. Brian: When the Levee Breaks," p. 176), the loss of her mucus plug, and/or having bloody show (blood vessels on the cervix begin to bleed as an indication of the cervix opening further) also suggest labor is close to beginning if it hasn't already and that it may be time to mobilize, or to sit back and continue waiting for the real thing to begin.

POTENTIAL PLOT TWISTS

Birthing isn't like professional wrestling, where outcomes are often predetermined. With such a vast array of variables involved in this production, predictability goes out the window. No two births are exactly alike. However, here are several of the most common developments you and your partner may encounter during the later stages of labor and delivery:

POPPING PANDORA'S BAG: THE AMNIOTOMY

If labor is especially slow-moving or if that lack of progress is threatening the health of the baby, the doctor may deem it time to intervene by rupturing the bag of waters, a move that not only allows medical personnel to see the color of the amniotic fluid (a means of determining whether the fetus is distressed), it also can induce or speed up

labor. Entering via the vagina, an instrument is used to put a hole in the amniotic sac. The amniotic fluid then begins to escape through that hole, usually leading to heightened labor activity.

A SHOT OF RELIEF: THE EPIDURAL

Roughly half the women who give birth in hospitals do so with the assistance of epidural anesthesia, in which painkilling or numbing drugs are introduced into the laboring woman's body, usually during active labor, to block pain in the lower part of her body. The anesthesia typically is administered by an anesthesiologist, a medical doctor who specializes in anesthesia, or a nurse-anesthetist, a nurse who also specializes in this particular procedure. If you find the sight of needles disturbing, you may want to avert your eyes during the procedure, because a needle will be inserted into your woman's lower back around the spinal cord (the epidural space), into which a catheter is carefully threaded through the needle. The needle is removed but the catheter remains to deliver more anesthesia as needed.

While an epidural blocks the lower body, it still may afford the woman freedom of movement, although she may be instructed not to walk about. Having an epidural should not prevent a woman from being awake and alert for the birth. Yet for a woman who's been laboring and in pain for many hours, having one can allow her to rest and gather strength before the final push.

Having an epidural relieves pain but it

also may make pushing more difficult due to the loss of feeling and may make an assisted birth necessary later in the process. And that numbness can linger for hours after she gives birth.

AIRLIFT: THE CESAREAN SECTION

A variety of conditions could prompt the medical team to determine a C-section must be performed. Dr. Brian describes this surgical procedure in detail on p. 196.

A STITCH IN TIME: THE EPISIOTOMY

Wonder why many women wince when they hear the word *episiotomy*? You'll cringe, too, when you learn what this procedure entails. Episiotomy is a surgical incision in the woman's perineum, the area between the vagina and rectum. The doctor may make such a cut during delivery to enlarge the vaginal opening for the baby to pass through, usually in instances when the baby's head is too large for the opening to accommodate, when the baby is in distress, or when the baby is in breech position. Immediately after birth, the incision is sutured. But it doesn't end there. Women who have had the procedure report that pain in the stitched area can linger and the healing can take several weeks or more. Here's where the caveman can help by leading his woman through Kegel exercises at least several times a week throughout pregnancy. In doing so, he's doing his part to keep the muscles in the area conditioned so she's better equipped to bounce back more quickly from an episiotomy or, better yet, to avoid the procedure altogether.

PULLED TO SAFETY: ASSISTED BIRTH

When the baby seems to have bottlenecked on his or her way down the birth canal and pushing no longer seems effective, it may be time for the doctor to reach into his toolbox for the forceps or vacuum extraction device. Forceps are an instrument that looks like spoon-shaped tongs. They are inserted into the vagina and opened to gently grasp both sides of the baby's head, around each cheek. The doctor then slowly guides the newborn through the last leg of the journey.

Vacuum extraction accomplishes the same thing, only using suction. Aided by light vacuum power, the funnel-shaped end of the device latches on to the top of baby's head via the vagina. The handle at the other end of the device is then used to coax the baby out into the waiting world.

Using forceps or a suction device can leave marks on the baby, but in the vast majority of cases those red areas and mild bruises disappear within a few days of birth. These devices also may contribute to the cone-shaped head some babies have at birth. Not to worry. The cone that is common to babies born vaginally rounds out in a few days.

HEAD'S UP: BREECH BIRTH

The optimal birthing position for a baby is head down, facing the woman's back. As birth approaches, however, a small percentage of babies end up in breech position, with their bottom or feet presenting first. There are several breech positions, including:

FRANK BREECH, which resembles the jackknife position, with the baby's butt pointed toward the birth canal, the legs in front of the body, and the feet up around the head

COMPLETE BREECH, which is more like a kneeling position, with the bottom down, legs folded at the knees, and feet tucked near the butt

FOOTLING BREECH, in which one or more of the baby's feet are poised to exit the woman first

Having a baby in breech position increases the likelihood a woman will have a cesarean section, assisted birth, and/or episiotomy.

THE FIRST STAGE OF LABOR

Contractions are gaining momentum, and what you calculated to be true after applying the 5-1-1 rule has been confirmed by a medical exam: your woman and you have officially entered the first stage of labor.

Labor's first stage is generally when your woman will experience most of her contractions. It actually unfolds in three phases: **early**, **active**, and **transition**, each typically more taxing on a woman than its predecessor. The early stage is considered the mellowest in terms of the demands it places on a woman, and thus at the suggestion of her medical provider, she may opt to spend part of labor's early phase at home, where she and her man can monitor contractions and try to stay relaxed in familiar surroundings.

What's happening down below at this point? The cervix typically is dilated to several centimeters in early labor. Contractions are coming regularly, their frequency varying from several minutes apart to fifteen or twenty minutes apart, depending on the person and the point to which labor has progressed.

Sometime during early labor (when the 5-1-1 rule dictates), you hopefully have made a move to your birthing location, because the time is approaching when your woman will need the labor and birthing squad to swing into action. If it's a particularly fast-moving labor, you may find yourselves arriving at the facility deeper into the process. With any luck, the process is not so far along that your child will be born outdoors as Gronk was.

Be prepared to support your woman in any manner possible, because the later phases of the first stage are when her uterus will do most of the hard contracting work—with the baby's help, of course. Your unborn child is much more than a bit player during labor, as he or she also must cooperate for all this to go smoothly. It is the position of the baby—preferably head down, facing mom's back—that largely determines how difficult labor and delivery will be. You will be counting on your *in utero* progeny to periodically adjust his or her position so it is optimal for heading head down the birthing canal. You'll also be relying on the baby to adjust positions while in the birthing canal to expedite that part of the journey.

For your woman, getting to the second stage of labor—the pushing and delivery stage—may be the most difficult and time-

DR. BRIAN

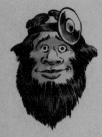

OOOH!
LOVE HURTS

I bring you pain
Pain makes you beautiful

—JUDYBATS,
"PAIN (MAKES YOU BEAUTIFUL)"

He is not a skilled reader of body language, but the expression the caveman sees on his woman's face tells him something serious is going down. It is the look of a primigravida who, for the first time, is experiencing the true contractions of labor. The Braxton-Hicks contractions she may have had periodically late in pregnancy were just light tremors compared with these temblors.

Usually brought on by a release of the hormone oxytocin, contractions are a tightening and relaxing of the uterine muscle. The uterus is the largest muscle in a woman's body, so when it contracts it tends to get attention. During labor, according to members of the Cultivated Caveman's Ad Hoc Female Advisory Council, contractions can start off as fairly tolerable—not too long, not too frequent, not too intense, a feeling akin to muscle cramping or gas pains. But the duration, frequency, and intensity of contractions can elevate unpredictably. That's when you are most likely to hear your woman roar.

A pregnant woman's body uses uterine contractions to push the fetus down toward and through the birth canal and pelvis. Contractions cause the cervix to dilate and efface, often growing more intense, more frequent, and longer as labor progresses (if you can call intense pain progress). Thankfully, even when contractions start coming rapidly and intensely, they do eventually come to an end, if only momentarily. This affords the heavily taxed woman a much-needed respite from the pain.

Oftentimes, our female sources concur, this pain is like nothing the woman has experienced before. This is when a woman may be most apt to collar a member of the birthing team and demand "meds" (such as an epidural injection) to ease her pain.

The look on your woman's face isn't the only indication she's in the midst of a contraction. If she lets you touch her abdomen during a contraction, you'll notice the muscles there are hard and taught as the fundus (the upper section of the uterus) tightens and thickens. This allows the lower part of the uterus to stretch and relax.

Contractions in the later phases of first-stage labor are usually the ones that register highest on the Richter scale. Each contraction reaches a peak before subsiding. As labor progresses, those peaks tend to come sooner and last longer.

Witnessing your woman endure this kind of discomfort can be harrowing. Your first instinct may be to protect her with some misguided act of chivalry. But remember, you are surrounded by people who have nothing but her best interests in mind. The most chivalrous thing you can do is bring her some water, massage her feet, back, or shoulders, or just offer words of encouragement and comfort. Here is where you stand aside and let your woman be the strong and invincible one.

STAGE 1 TO-DO LIST FOR THE CAN-DO CAVEMAN

BLOODY (GOOD) SHOW: prepare yourself for graphic viewing—blood, body cavities, the works.

BE HER CADDY, suggesting position shifts and helping her shift into them, reminding her to empty her bladder periodically, offering comforting words, sharing the excitement and nerves of the moment.

REMIND YOURSELF but do not verbalize the fact that women's bodies are built for childbirth, contrary to what appears possible to the naked caveman eye.

HELP HER PASS THE TIME by engaging her in conversation (if she's up for talking), playing some of her favorite music on the stereo, playing cards, watching television, and taking occasional walks and a bath or shower, whatever relieves her and helps the minutes pass faster.

OFFER LIGHT FOOD AND DRINK, provided you have cleared it with members of the medical staff.

START YOUR MASSAGE ACTIVITY to help her relax and to address spots where she's feeling the most pain or discomfort.

If your birthing strategy calls for the use of **BREATHING TECHNIQUES,** start using them as needed.

USE VISUALIZATION TECHNIQUES in which the woman mentally envisions the cervix opening and the baby moving into and through the opening.

HER WISH IS YOUR COMMAND: provide cool towels, lip balm, and whatever else she needs.

ENCOURAGE YOUR WOMAN to resist the urge to push. Save that for the second stage.

DON YOUR SCRUBS if you are truly committed to looking the part and "playing doctor."

TURN OFF YOUR CELL PHONE and do not turn it back on until cleared by mom.

consuming part of the process. Indeed, labor's first stage can last anywhere from a few hours to fifteen hours or more. If she begins showing signs of wear or impatience, try consoling her by pointing out that she likely will spend the most time in this first phase, when contractions are considered mildest. If she reacts venomously, sarcastically, or indifferently to your point, she may well have advanced to active labor, the second phase of the first stage. This is when labor pains tend to increase as contractions become longer and closer together, coming roughly every few minutes and causing your woman to show increasing signs of discomfort—backache, muscle cramps, etc. The more intense contractions also are doing their work to open the cervix, which at this point in active labor is dilated to the four- to seven-centimeter range.

The needle on the contraction intensity gauge, already climbing during the active phase, really jumps in the last phase of first-stage labor, called transition labor. The baby is heading down to the lower reaches of the uterus now, causing intensifying, longer, and more frequent contractions. If her water hasn't broken yet, it probably will at some point in this phase.

If you are ever going to hear your woman roar, this will be the time. Contractions during the transition phase are typically of a greater magnitude than any of their predecessors, lasting a minute to a minute and a half, with pauses of just a couple minutes in between. While transition typically is the shortest phase of first-stage labor, it may

seem like the longest. For first-time mothers, it can last several hours, while for mothers who have had a vaginal delivery before, the process typically goes quicker.

Here's where the laboring woman can be stricken with nausea, vomiting, acute backache, heavy show, rectal pressure, cramps, and other symptoms. It's also when the caveman finds out about his threshold for graphic viewing. It's no wonder that most females who have been through the process report that transition labor can't end fast enough. Mercifully, it will come to an end. The first stage is officially over when the numbers read like this: cervix 100-percent effaced and dilated to ten centimeters. Time to begin pushing—onward to Stage 2.

THE SECOND STAGE OF LABOR

So help me, please, doctor, I'm damaged
You can put back my heart in its hole
Oh mama, I'm cryin'
Tears of relief
And my pulse is now under control
—THE ROLLING STONES, "DEAR DOCTOR"

Now the numbers on the labor scoreboard indicate your woman has officially made it to the second stage of labor—the Red Zone. If things go according to plan, much of the hard work is behind her, and parenthood looms just ahead. Labor's second stage typically is much shorter than the first, lasting a matter of minutes to an hour or two and

DR. BRIAN

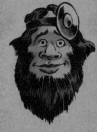

THE LABORING WOMAN'S MEDICINE CHEST

....

This felt a lot better going in than it does coming out!

—QUOTE FROM LABORING
PATIENT OF DR. BRIAN'S AS
HER BABY IS CROWNING

....

An expectant mother may require various drugs during labor and delivery to speed the process, slow it down, or make it less painful, as dictated by her preferences and her condition. The caveman may want a stash of his own, but his job is to stay lucid. Don't be surprised if in the throes of labor your woman curses you, the prehistoric impregnator, for your role in putting her in a family way. Don't discourage her if she demands pain medication such as an epidural, even if in your birthing plan you specify a "natural childbirth," free of painkilling drugs. Childbirth is not an endurance test, so taking something to dull the pain should not be regarded as a failure. Look at it this way: if men were the ones giving birth, morphine drips would be mandatory and the birth rate would plummet to an all-time low. Here's a look at several medications the doctor may recommend:

▶ **NARCOTICS** such as Demerol may be used to mask pain in the early stages of labor.

▶ **AN EPIDURAL BLOCK** is often administered to ease pain during active labor. This is a narcotic (pain-masking) and anesthetic (pain-blocking) cocktail that is injected into a space surrounding the spinal nerves. Having what's called a "walking epidural" may allow her to walk during labor.

▶ **THE SPINAL BLOCK,** like an epidural block, is a mixture of anesthetic and narcotic. Often used with a cesarean birth, this one renders her with virtually no feeling from the chest down.

▶ **LOCAL ANESTHESIA,** including chloroprocaine, lidocaine, and other "-caines" are administered locally into the tissue of the vagina, usually before an episiotomy or to repair a tear in the tissue.

▶ **INDUCTION DRUGS,** such as prostaglandins or a synthetic form of the hormone oxytocin, are used when the doctor deems it necessary to jumpstart labor. Usually this happens when a woman is past her delivery due date, because it is in the fetus's best health interests and/or because the expectant mother has a condition such as preeclampsia, diabetes, etc. Synthetic oxytocin (Pitocin) is administered via an IV drip.

▶ If a woman goes into labor prematurely, she's apt to be given some form of a **TOCOLYTIC MEDICATION** to stop or slow the process.

culminating with the event you have been working toward for the past nine months or more: the birth of your child. For the three of you, there is light at the end of the tunnel.

As transition labor yields to second-stage labor, many women will enjoy a brief respite from contractions. Once the breather ends and contractions resume, they may slow to as much as five minutes apart, with a duration of sixty to ninety seconds. This is also when the woman's persistent urge to push becomes almost uncontrollable with each contraction. Finally she will be allowed to answer that urge, pushing during contractions to direct the baby down the birthing canal.

It may take awhile for your woman to find her optimal position for the birth. Several positions are commonly used to allow the baby to exit, including side-lying, sitting propped up in a semi-inclined position, squatting, and on all fours, with weight on her hands and knees. In many cases the positioning of the baby will dictate which birthing position she finds most comfortable and conducive to a safe exit for the baby.

Eventually the baby's head will drop down so low it may apply extreme pressure on her rectum. When the head passes through the vagina, it is considered to be in crowning position. If you have the fortitude and permission to look down there, crowning is when you may catch your first glimpse of the baby's head.

The woman's chosen birthing position is perhaps the foremost of several factors that determine how the caveman positions him-

PONDER THIS

THINGS NOT TO DO IN THE DELIVERY ROOM

Some of your usual behaviors must be modified during the minutes, hours, or days you spend with Mrs. Gronk in the delivery room. A general rule of thumb is allow her to be the general and be as solicitous, polite, and obedient as a buck private. Here is a simple list of orders. Do not:

▶ **EAT ANY PUNGENT FOOD,** especially of the onion, garlic, bbq-flavored variety (women in labor tend to be hypersensitive to odors of any kind)

▶ **MAKE ANY REMARKS** whatsoever about female genitalia

▶ **WATCH TV** excessively

▶ **EXCLAIM** "Oh my God," "Holy shit," "Guh-ross"

▶ **HIT ON MEDICAL STAFF**

▶ **BURY HEAD** in the sports page or other reading material

▶ **TALK ON CELL PHONE** or use other handheld communications devices

▶ **ACT NONPLUSSED,** with frequent glances at watch

▶ **SURF THE WEB**

▶ **BECOME ATTACHED** to iPod

▶ **OBSTRUCT** other members of the labor and delivery team

▶ **VOMIT**

▶ **PASS OUT**

self during the birthing process. You want to be in a position that will:

- Afford you access to your woman, so you can offer words of encouragement and comfort and respond to her requests

- Put you within reach of areas to massage her

- Allow you to see only as much as you want to see

- Allow you to hold one of your woman's legs during pushing if you are prepared or asked to do so

- Give you the chance to cut the baby's umbilical cord, if you are prepared or asked to do so

- Allow you to temporarily step away and steady yourself if what you are seeing makes your stomach churn or head swim

While the caveman concerns himself with finding an optimal position, his woman has larger, more painful concerns—namely the baby's head. As the largest part of the baby's body, the head usually is the most painful for a woman to push through. When the baby is crowning, the doctor may deem it necessary to perform an episiotomy, an incision in the perineum that opens the birth canal more broadly for the baby to pass. Here's another moment when your staying power and stomach for graphic viewing may be severely tested. While a guy may want no part of viewing these espe-

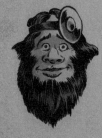

DR. BRIAN

EMERGENCY EXIT: THE CESAREAN SECTION

History is full of men whose actions and deeds make them role models for the cultivated cavemen of today. Julius Caesar, who ruled a far-reaching empire during the first century BC, was such a man. A brilliant tactician, powerful leader, and architect of the Roman Empire, Caesar conquered exotic lands and exotic women, even siring a son with Cleopatra, the beautiful and mysterious queen of Egypt. And through it all, he wore a toga.

Not only will your woman don a modern version of the toga—a birthing gown—during childbirth, she also may encounter a reminder of Caesar's empire, the cesarean section. The C-section is a procedure named for none other than Julius Caesar himself, who, according to historical accounts, was surgically removed from his mother's womb around 100 BC. In performing the technique today, a doctor makes an incision in the pregnant woman's abdomen and lifts the baby out through the uterus. Here in the twenty-first century, C-sections occur more frequently than one might imagine. They accounted for 29.1 percent of the 4.1 million baby deliveries in the United States in 2004, an all-time high, according to the U.S. Centers for Disease Control and Prevention. And if a woman delivers her first child by cesarean (these days more than one in four first-timers do), CDC statistics say she has close to a 90 percent chance of delivering subsequent children that way.

Typically the procedure lasts less than an hour, while the woman is under some form of anesthesia (such as an epidural). So while she may be awake during the surgery, she won't feel the initial vertical or horizontal abdominal incision nor the subsequent uterine incision. Having gained entry into the uterus, the surgeon uses a device to drain the amniotic fluid, then lifts the baby out to meet his or her makers. Next the placenta is lifted out as well, after which the incisions are closed with sutures.

Doctors recommend women have cesarean sections for a range of reasons, some of the most common of which are listed below. Keep in mind, just because your woman has one or more of these conditions does not guarantee she will need a C-section.

- The woman has placenta previa, a condition in which the placenta is obstructing the cervix.

- The woman has a placental abruption, in which her placenta prematurely separates from the uterine lining.

- The woman has a tear or rupture in her uterus.

- The fetus is in breech position, its legs or butt presenting down the birth canal instead of the head.

- There is a cord prolapse, in which the position of the umbilical cord diminishes blood flow to the baby.

- The fetus is in distress because of a lack of oxygen or some other cause.

- Labor fails to progress, such as if the cervix has not fully dilated or if labor started then slowed or stopped.

- The baby's positioning is problematic, such as with a breech presentation.

- A cephalopelvic disproportion (CPD) has been diagnosed, indicating either the baby's head is too large or the mother's pelvis is too small for a vaginal birth.

- The woman has active genital herpes, has developed gestational diabetes, or is a diabetic.

- The woman has been diagnosed with preeclampsia—high blood pressure during pregnancy.

- It's a multiple birth (more than one child).

In a perfect world, most expectant parents and their medical providers would choose a vaginal birth over a C-section, mainly because of the risks posed by the surgery and the major impact the procedure has on a woman's body. A vaginal birth can be long and painful, but the recovery from a cesarean section tends to be much more lengthy. Still, some women voluntarily choose to have a C-section.

Since a C-section is considered major surgery, there are risks associated with it: infection, blood loss, blood clots, and other unsavory but remote possibilities. The vast majority of cesarean births go smoothly and the two key parties involved, mother and child, emerge healthy.

Knowing what the surgery entails, many cavemen choose not to watch as it unfolds, instead positioning themselves so their view of this especially graphic scene is obstructed. If your woman appears destined for a C-section—some couples know well in advance that this is how their child will be born—and you feel absolutely certain you want to view the entire procedure up-close, you'll want to first clear it with your medical team, then spend some time watching the Surgery Channel to build tolerance.

STAGE 2 TO-DO LIST FOR THE CAN-DO CAVEMAN

HELP HER CHANGE POSITIONS to find one she likes best for birthing.

REASSURE YOURSELF but do not verbalize the fact that a woman's vagina is a highly elastic and resilient organ, that it will make it through this experience relatively intact, despite what appears to be one of those bowling-ball-through-a-garden-hose scenarios.

COACH HER through the pushing by pacing her breathing.

KEEP HER IN RHYTHM by counting through each push.

If she wants a **MASSAGE,** give her one. If she wants you to **HOLD HER HAND,** do it.

KEEP YOUR COMPOSURE.

If you feel queasy, **STAND BACK, TAKE A SEAT FOR A MOMENT** so you don't obstruct other members of the medical team, and once you feel stable again, **RETURN TO YOUR POST.**

HAVE A MIRROR READY so she has the option of watching the baby emerge from the birthing canal.

HAVE A CAMERA READY to capture the first still or action footage of the first meeting between baby and mom.

cially graphic developments, the woman at this point may ask for a mirror so she can see the goings-on.

This is typically when the attending doctor makes an appearance to facilitate the baby's final thrust to glory. Here comes the head. Now the shoulders, waist, and rest of the body exit. Though bodily fluids cover much of the wrinkled newborn's body, one glimpse in the area of the genitals tells you it's clearly a…

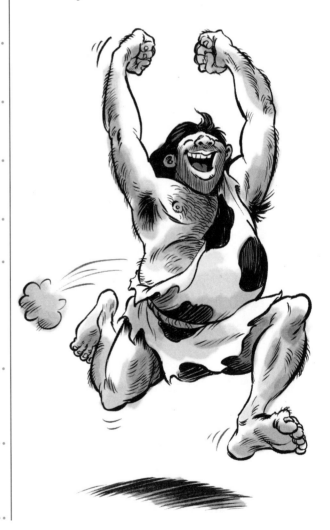

THE THIRD STAGE OF LABOR

It ain't over till it's over.

—YOGI BERRA

Congratulations are again in order, just as they were many long weeks ago, when you first found out for sure the two of you were expecting. Now you have earned the right to call yourselves parents. After all this work, you and your woman, exhausted, trembling, and ecstatic, finally get to hold Baby Unibrow.

Even the most stoic of cavemen may need to reach for a handkerchief when he watches his woman hold the caveling on her chest for the first time. Let her bask in the glow of motherhood for a few minutes as she holds the baby, then reach for the camera to capture this moving moment on film. Humor her if she demands you brush her hair prior to snapping any photos.

Once this moment passes, and before you run out to light a cigar or pop a bottle of champagne in triumph, there is a bit more work to be done—relatively minor, but work nonetheless. So while you are holding the baby or handing the newborn over to the nurses to deal with cleanup and other postpartum activities, your woman must continue pushing for a short period of time to deliver the now-vacant bag of waters and the placenta, which should have separated from the walls of the uterus after the baby's birth. This rather anticlimactic last act of labor,

STAGE 3 TO-DO LIST FOR THE CAN-DO CAVEMAN

CRY IF YOU FEEL LIKE CRYING, shout if you feel like shouting, dance if you feel like dancing.

With doctor's permission, **SEE THAT MOM GETS TO HOLD BABY** immediately after birth.

GRAB A CAMERA to capture the first moments of baby's life and mom's first meeting with the newcomer.

Once cleared by medical personnel, **BRING THE NEWBORN OUT** to meet any awaiting friends and family.

TURN ON CELL PHONE and start spreading the news.

PREPARE CELEBRATORY ITEMS: cigar, champagne, etc.

known as delivering the afterbirth, usually lasts no more than thirty minutes. The placenta is a blood-rich organ, so consider yourself warned: seeing it delivered is not a sight for a caveman with a weak constitution.

PLEASED TO MEET YOU

*Ain't nobody knows what the newborn
   holds
But his mama says he'll walk on water
And wander back home*

—IRON & WINE,
"FREEDOM HANGS LIKE HEAVEN"

Even the wailing Ice Age wind that blows across the desolate tundra cannot drown out the joyful exclamations and shrieks that emanate from the mouth of the cave this Paleolithic evening. The racket comes from a rejoicing clan of Cro-Magnons as they welcome another member and celebrate the survival of both mother and healthy newborn. Childbirth was an especially risky proposition back then, but this time it has gone exceedingly well.

His adrenaline still pumping following the birth, one clan member triumphantly brandishes the newborn above his head for all in the cave to see. He is a first-time father at the ripe old age of seventeen. Meanwhile, a female several years his junior lies spent in a bed of animal pelts, a smile on her flushed face. She is the mother. This is their first child together and later they will celebrate by making an offering of the expelled amniotic sac and placenta to the gods of health and fertility.

A similar but modernized version of this celebration is underway in your birthing suite following the birth of your child. You have a pretty clear vision of what your next steps are: start distributing cigars, making phone calls, and pouring the champagne. But what about the stars of the show, the new mom and newborn?

Here in the postpartum or neonatal phase, mother and baby both will be watched closely. After a sometimes uncomfortable nine months getting acclimated to pregnancy, your woman now must quickly reverse fields and readjust to not being pregnant. Within the first hour or two after birth, her vital signs will be monitored closely to spot potential complications. As for the baby, he or she likely will be placed under a heat source, tested for health, cleaned of the substances that attached themselves to him or her in the womb and birthing canal, and swaddled for warmth, then brought to the nursery.

Before that trip to the nursery, the two of you have a golden opportunity to get to know your offspring. It's never too early to begin bonding with the newborn. In fact, studies have shown that interacting with the baby right after birth may lead to a tighter bond. This is not to suggest the caveman dad initiate a one-sided discussion of sports, curfew time, or dating guidelines, only that he hold and speak to the newcomer, perhaps offering a lullaby as well. It is in these early moments that mothers in most cases will be encouraged to try to breast-feed the newborn, another key step in the bonding process, but one you can only observe.

Within a few hours of birth, once your

woman has stabilized and if there are no complications, the postpartum nursing team takes over for the labor and delivery nursing team. They will be the ones who care for your woman and child through the end of your hospital stay. They will attend to your woman, focusing their efforts on the often-ravaged pelvic area, particularly if the birth involved an episiotomy or there was tearing of the vaginal tissue.

But what's happening with the new arrival? Hospital maternity wards have nurseries where newborns spend much of their time before going home with their parents. Nurses will attend to them there and bring them to mom when it's time to breast-feed or just to spend some quality time together. Many hospitals allow parents to choose between having their child stay in the nursery or in the room with his or her parents. In many cases a woman who has just given birth opts for the former so she can enjoy some uninterrupted sleep after labor and delivery, knowing she can ask a nurse to bring the baby to her anytime.

The postpartum period provides the caveman with another excellent opportunity to practice using more of his new vocabulary words, including:

JAUNDICE: A common condition that can give the baby's skin a yellowish tint

BILIRUBIN: A substance in the blood that can build up and cause jaundice

LOCHIA: Liquid that flows from a woman's vagina following childbirth

DR. BRIAN

YOUR BABY'S FIRST TEST (NO. 2 PENCIL NEEDED)

Your baby is out of the womb only a few moments, and already as parents you're worrying about test scores—not standardized school tests or the SATS but what's called the APGAR test, which measures how your newborn is doing at one minute past birth and again at five minutes past birth. The APGAR test grades newborns on a scale of one to ten, ten being a rare perfect score. APGAR is an acronym for the five areas in which the baby's health and well-being are rated:

- ➤ **A**ctivity/muscle tone
- ➤ **P**ulse
- ➤ **G**rimace response/reflex irritability
- ➤ **A**ppearance/skin color
- ➤ **R**espiration

Nurses and doctors examine the baby and assign a score of up to two points in each of those five categories. A baby who scores seven or more on the first-minute test is generally considered to be in good health, though a score below seven doesn't necessarily indicate something is wrong, only that the newborn may need extra attention (supplementary oxygen, clearing of the air passage) and a few minutes to stabilize. That's why the APGAR score is calculated again at five minutes. At that point, if a newborn still scores below a seven, he or she may need additional care, treatment, and monitoring by the medical staff.

LACTATION: The woman's production of milk

ENGORGEMENT: After birth, when a woman's breasts first fill with milk

SUCKING REFLEX: The baby's instinct to search for the breast in a quest for mother's milk; known still to be present in most full-grown cavemen

MASTITIS: A breast infection that afflicts some new mothers

MECONIUM: The greenish-black, tarlike substance that typically comprises the baby's first bowel movement

COLOSTRUM: The thick, yellowish liquid produced by a woman's breasts as the precursor to milk; the baby will feed on this protein-rich substance for several days, until mom's milk comes in

COLIC: A condition in which a newborn cries for long stretches with no apparent cause. Pray it doesn't happen to you.

THREE A.M. FEEDING: Who eats at that hour? Club-hoppers and partygoers do. So do newborns.

LOW BIRTHWEIGHT

According to the National Center for Health Statistics (NCHS), a low birthweight baby weighs less than 5 pounds, 8 ounces at birth and a very low birthweight infant weighs less than 3 pounds, 4 ounces. Low birthweight can be a serious situation for a newborn trying to make it in the outside world. Most low birthweight and virtually all very low birthweight babies are born prior to full term. About 8 percent of all

babies born in the U.S. are termed low birthweight and about 1.5 percent as very low birthweight. These babies have to quickly make up the weight that they may have gained tucked away in the womb. The nurses will weigh your baby very soon after delivery and will let you know your newborn's weight. If there are concerns about the baby's heft, the newborn will need to stay in the hospital to fatten up.

HASTA LA VISTA, BABY

Now you can talk the talk and walk the walk of a new parent. But y'all can't go home just yet (unless it was a home birth, obviously), because both baby and mother are in a relatively fragile postpartum state. Both need to rest and regain their strength. Chances are your woman is going be wobbly after all she's been through emotionally and physically. She is going to need time to recuperate in the hospital (if that's where the birth occurred), then more time to heal and recoup strength at home. If she has given birth vaginally, her stay in the hospital will last a day or two after birth. If the baby was born by C-section, she could be in the hospital for up to a week, with more recuperation to come at home as well.

It's called a hospital, but the brand of hospitality served up in the facility's postpartum wing caters more to the infant and new mom than to the cavedad. Unless, of course, your idea of comfort is a vinyl-upholstered pull-out couch for sleeping, cafeteria-crafted "food" for dinner, and frequent middle-of-

CHECKOUT TIME

Hospitals and other birthing venues have policies about just when mother and child may go their merry way. Some have early-departure options of 12 hours, while others make it a minimum of 24. It's best to check ahead with your spot to be prepared about how long after the birth your family needs to stick around.

the-night intrusions by medical staff. If so, you're never going to want the postpartum hospital stay to end! This isn't the case with every venue, but be prepared.

In most hospitals and birthing centers, new dads are welcome to stay overnight with their partner and baby in the postpartum wing. This area is often its own little insular world, where parents and newborns can relish their first hours and days together as a family unit, largely apart from real world distractions. The surroundings may be spartan, but the time spent in the hospital after the birth of your child is precious and worth savoring, even if the food isn't.

Be prepared to endure a seemingly non-stop procession of medical visits, from the pediatrician's examination of the newborn and a follow-up from the OB-GYN and/or midwife to frequent appearances by nurses to monitor mom's condition (blood pressure,

body temperature, and a peek beneath the gown to see how her reproductive organs are recovering). Depending on the hospital or birthing facility, there may also be visits by a lactation consultant (to help your woman with breast-feeding if she needs it), plus opportunities for new parents to sit in on classes right in the nursery to learn about such practicalities as how to hold, bottle-feed, burp, and diaper a baby.

During your hopefully brief postpartum hospital stay, there will be many real-world intrusions. Between moments of blissed-out joy and exhaustion, you'll have to submit to some duties and interruptions, but this is where you can shine. Commit to these tasks and interactions with humor and patience and your good vibes will transfer to your new family.

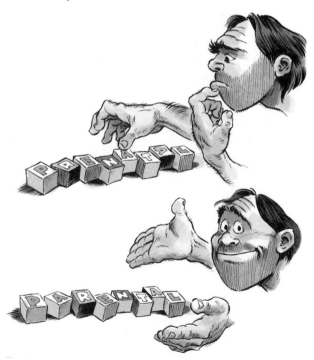

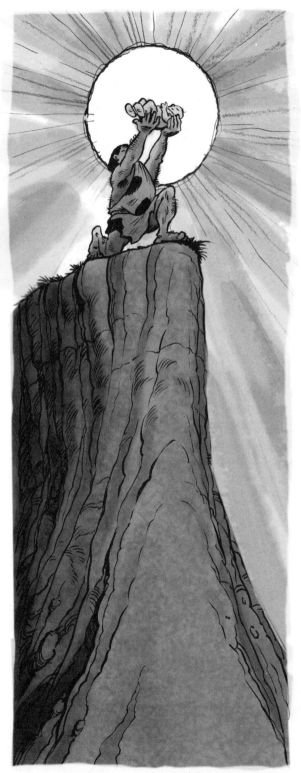

POSTPARTUM POSTERBOY: LIFE AS A CULTIVATED CAVEDAD

Welcome to the postpartum party, pops. Like pregnancy, parenthood is another new frontier, full of surprises both beautiful and terrifying. Anxious? Excited? Scared? Intimidated? Ecstatic? You will have good reason to be all those. The delivery of your child is the rite of passage that officially vaults you and your woman from the we-first phase of life to the wee-one-first phase of life. For first-time parents, this is all-new territory.

Take heart, because a healthy newborn baby is resilient and built to function well in the outside world. But that doesn't mean the

POSTPARTUM PAPERWORK

Believe it or not, you should apply for a Social Security number for the baby right away, so he or she can enjoy all the wonderful benefits Uncle Sam bestows upon enrollees. It's part of the birth registration process in hospitals and birthing centers and takes about five weeks for you to receive the number. The birthing facility itself and your insurance company will also have multiple forms for you to fill out. Have your number two pencil sharpened and ready, my man.

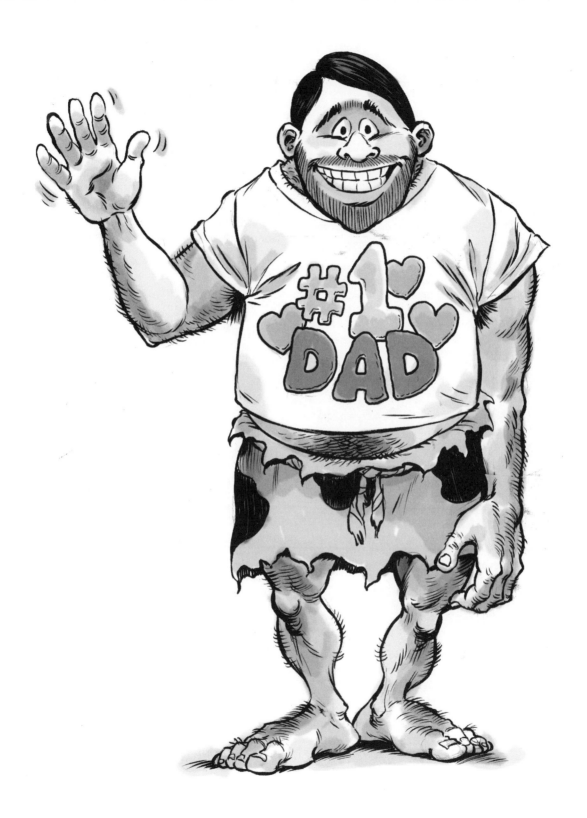

PONDER THIS

PARTING WISDOM FOR
THE POSTPARTUM PERIOD

The parental head-scratching begins virtually from the moment your new child is born. Here are a few pointers for new dads:

▶ Remember her emotional ups and downs during pregnancy? Expect more of the same during the postpartum period, when some women may get the blues (or even depression) as their hormones seek out their pre-pregnancy levels, and as the anticipation and excitement of pregnancy and birth yield to the realities of life as a parent. New dads also can get the postpartum blues.

▶ Sleep may come sporadically and sparingly for expectant parents, so grab catnaps whenever you can. When the infant sleeps, try to catch some shut-eye yourself.

▶ For a newborn who is having trouble sleeping, try putting a T-shirt that bears mom's scent in the youngster's cradle or sleeping area. Babies rely heavily on their olfactory sense, so the familiar scent of mom and her milk could put the newborn at ease.

▶ The milk in the small, plastic bottle is the richest-tasting, most nutritious in the fridge. But hands off—this is breast milk your woman has worked hard to pump for the baby, it's not for you to drop in your cereal or coffee. If you are that curious about tasting it, ask for a sip directly from the tap.

▶ Hold on and hold out, cowboy. Just because your woman has given birth doesn't mean she can jump right back on the proverbial hobbyhorse. Her doctor, her body, and her emotional state, not your wanton urges, will dictate when it's ok to resume sexual intercourse. In most cases it takes between four and six weeks for a woman to heal from a vaginal birth and perhaps longer to bounce back from a cesarean section. Until then, rely on your private movie collection and ride one-handed for a while.

▶ Give yourselves a breather from the visitor parade. As exhausting as it is to go through labor and delivery, it's great to have friends and family around right after the birth. You can show off the new arrival and they can help around the house as the two of you get accustomed to your new parental duties. But there's a fine line between having enough help and having too many visitors. New parents need time with the baby and moments to savor the new family structure by themselves, free from visitors. So do your best to schedule accordingly, at the risk of roiling your mother-in-law.

youngster comes out of the womb equipped to join you in the hunt or to forage for his or her own food. The helpless youth will rely on the shelter, warmth, nourishment, care and safety you provide. And now, you are eminently equipped to be a provider. You'll have to wait a few months before you begin cooking the newcomer some of your caveman culinary specialties (have a good recipe for mush?), but right away you can get busy strumming lullabies for the little one on your guitar or knitting the newcomer a blanket or winter cap-and-scarf set.

This is where you and your mentor Gronk must part ways, at least for now. The intrepid caveman Gronk has his own family to attend to, so he'll be prevented from holding your hand through the next stage of life. Not that you need any handholding at this juncture, for having persevered through pregnancy and childbirth, you have proven your mettle and your ability to adapt and thrive in unfamiliar environments. You have turned yourself into a true cultivated caveman, one who possesses many of the qualities necessary to survive and thrive as a parent. For you to have come this far in the evolutionary process in such a short time is a harbinger of good things to come for you as a father and for the three of you as a family.

As a proud new papa and cultivated caveman, you have indeed kissed the Stone Age goodbye. New horizons of cultivation await you as a parent. So grab your little family and venture forth from the cave, young man. The twenty-first century beckons.

RESOURCES

There is a vast amount of information available for the modern caveman and his fairer partner about pregnancy and childbirth. Here is a brief selection of resources for expectant parents to explore along the path to parenthood and beyond. None of the information in these sources is a substitution for a consultation with a professional health care provider. Find qualified people whose judgment you trust and call upon them to help you with questions about your specific situation.

WEBSITES

American Academy of Family Physicians (AAFP): www.aafp.org

American Association of Birth Centers: www.birthcenters.org

American College of Nurse-Midwives: www.midwife.org

American College of Obstetricians and Gynecologists (ACOG): www.acog.org

American Diabetes Association: www.diabetes.org/gestational-diabetes.jsp

American Dietetic Association: www.eatright.org

American Heart Association: www.americanheart.org

American Lung Association: www.lungusa.org

American Pregnancy Association: www.americanpregnancy.org

American Red Cross: www.redcross.org.

Canavan Research Foundation: www.canavan.org

Colic: www.mayoclinic.com/health/colic/DS00058

Cardiopulmonary Resuscitation (CPR): www.depts.washington.edu/learncpr/infantcpr.html

Circumcision: www.familydoctor.org, search "circumcision"

Cystic Fibrosis Foundation: www.cff.org

Doulas of North America (DONA): www.dona.org

March of Dimes: www.marchofdimes.com/pnhec/pnhec.asp

Midwives Alliance of North America (MANA): www.mana.org

National Down Syndrome Society: www.ndss.org

National Institutes of Health (NIH): www.nih.org

National Marrow Donor Program, Cord Blood: www.marrow.org/nmdp/center_for_cb.html

National Organization of Rare Diseases: www.rarediseases.org

National Tay-Sachs and Allied Diseases: www.ntsad.org

National Women's Health Information Center: www.4woman.gov

Sickle Cell Disease Association of America: www.sicklecelldisease.org

U.S.F.D.A., Seafood Information Resources: http://www.cfsan.fda.gov/seafood1.html

U.S. Centers for Disease Control and Prevention (CDC): www.cdc.gov

BOOKS

Belly Laughs (Da Capo, 2004) by Jenny McCarthy

The Birth Book (Little, Brown, 1994) by William Sears, M.D. and Martha Sears, R.N.

A Child Is Born (Delta, 2004) by Lennart Nilsson

The Complete Book of Pregnancy and Childbirth (Knopf, 2003) by Sheila Kitzinger

The Complete Kama Sutra (Diane Publishing, 2001) translated by Alain Daniélou

Eating for Pregnancy (Collins, 2004) by Catherine Jones

Eating Expectantly (Meadowbrook, 2000) by Bridget Swinney, M.S., R.D.

The Expectant Father (Abbeville, 2001) by Armin A. Brott and Jennifer Ash

The Girlfriends' Guide to Pregnancy (Pocket, 1995) by Vicki Iovine

Mayo Clinic Guide to a Healthy Pregnancy (Collins, 2004) edited by Roger W. Harms, M.D.

Natural Childbirth the Bradley Way (Plume, 1996) by Susan McCutcheon

Planning Your Pregnancy and Birth, Third Edition (American College of Obstetricians and Gynecologists, 2001) by American College of Obstetricians and Gynecologists

The Pregnancy Book (Little, Brown, 1997) by William Sears, M.D. and Martha Sears, R.N.

The Pregnancy Cookbook (W. W. Norton, 2002) by Hope Ricciotini, M.D. and Vincent Connelly

Your Baby and Child (Knopf, 1997) by Penelope Leach

Your Pregnancy Week by Week, Fifth Edition (Da Capo, 2004) by Glade B. Curtis and Judith Schuler

GLOSSARY

A

ACTIVE LABOR. Second phase of the first stage of labor, when contractions become longer, more frequent, and intense.

ALPHA-FETOPROTEIN (AFP). Part of the second trimester screening, which is used to assess the risk of Down Syndrome, Trisomy 18, and neural tube defects, including spina bifida and anencephaly.

AFTERBIRTH. Empty amniotic sac and placenta, delivered by (or extracted from) a woman after birth.

AMNIOCENTESIS. Medical procedure, usually performed between 16–20 weeks of pregnancy, in which amniotic fluid and cells are extracted from the amniotic sac within the pregnant woman's uterus, then analyzed to identify fetal genetic health.

AMNIOTIC FLUID. Fluid in the amniotic sac, surrounding the fetus for protection; supply of the fluid is frequently replenished. As it can be an indicator of fetal health, the amount of amniotic fluid may be monitored.

AMNIOTIC SAC. Thin membrane filled with amniotic fluid (and the placenta) that serves as a fetal shock absorber.

AMNIOTOMY. Procedure in which the amniotic sac is purposely punctured in order to start or speed labor.

ANESTHESIA. Drugs administered to a patient to block and mask pain during a medical procedure. General anesthesia renders a patient unconscious; local anesthesia removes feeling from a portion of the body.

ANESTHESIOLOGIST. Medical doctor specializing in the delivery of anesthesia.

ANTEPARTUM. The period of time when a woman is pregnant.

APGAR TEST. Method to measure how a newborn is faring just after birth, with a one-to-ten scoring scale; acronym for the five areas in which the baby's health and well-being are rated: Activity/muscle tone; Pulse; Grimace response/reflex irritability; Appearance/skin color; Respiration.

ASSISTED BIRTH. When a baby is delivered with the help of forceps or vacuum device.

B

BILIRUBIN. Normally occurring substance in the blood that in a newborn can reach higher-than-normal levels, causing jaundice.

BIRTHING ASSISTANT. See doula

BIRTHING PLAN. Written plan explaining expectations and specifications for labor and delivery.

BLOODY SHOW. Bleeding as a result of the opening of the cervix in preparation for and during labor.

BRAXTON-HICKS CONTRACTIONS. Known as false, or practice, contractions, usually irregularly timed and less intense than true labor contractions.

BREECH (POSITION). When a baby's buttocks, or one or both legs, is nearer to the birth canal, rather than the head. Frequently requires delivery by cesarean section.

BREAST PUMP. Manual or powered device that gently pumps milk from the breast of a lactating woman.

C

CALCIUM. Nutrient that fosters fetal formation of strong bones and teeth.

CANAVAN DISEASE. Genetically inherited fatal disorder of the brain and nervous system. Most common among Ashkenazi Jewish populations; cvs and amniocentesis can detect the disease prior to birth.

CARDIOPULMONARY RESUSCITATION (CPR). Method using timed compression and breathing to revive a person in cardiac and/or respiratory arrest.

CARDIOVASCULAR EXERCISE. Sustained activity to raise the heart and respiratory rates; also called "cardio."

CEPHALOPELVIC DISPROPORTION (CPD). When a baby's head is too large to fit through a woman's pelvis and vaginal opening during birth.

CERVIX. Lowest section of the uterus.

CESAREAN SECTION (CESAREAN BIRTH). Surgical delivery a baby through the abdominal wall, also called "C-section."

CHANGING TABLE. Furniture topped by a flat, washable surface for changing a baby's diapers and clothes.

CIRCUMCISION. Surgical removal of the foreskin of the penis.

COLIC. Condition in which a baby cries for extended periods of time with no apparent cause.

COLOSTRUM. Fluid, typically light yellow or milky white in color, secreted by a woman's breasts during the end of, and just after, pregnancy.

CONCEPTION. Successful fertilization of an egg by a sperm.

CONTRACTION. Rhythmic cycle in which the uterine muscles tighten and shorten, then relax; may occur before labor (Braxton-Hicks contractions) but the onset of regular contractions usually indicates labor has begun. The muscle action of contractions helps position the fetus for delivery.

CONTRAINDICATION. When it is inadvisable to use a particular medication or procedure, or to take part in a particular activity.

CORD PROLAPSE. When the umbilical cord passes into the birth canal before the baby, so that the delivering baby will put pressure to the cord, cutting off it's own blood flow and oxygen. Usually an obstetric emergency requiring emergency C-section.

COUVADE. Psychosomatic condition of males who experience sympathetic conditions including nausea and body aches during a mate's pregnancy.

CRO-MAGNON. Early form of human that lived from about 35,000 to 10,000 years ago.

CROSS-CONTAMINATION. Contaminating food with bacteria or other potentially harmful substance by lack of proper kitchen safety practices.

CROWNING. During labor, when the baby's head reaches the opening of the vagina.

CYSTIC FIBROSIS. Genetically inherited disease effecting the pulmonary and digestive systems. Most common among Caucasian and Northern European populations; cvs and amniocentesis can detect the disease prior to birth.

D

DIETARY SUPPLEMENT(S). Nutrients other than food taken during pregnancy.

DILATION. When the cervix opens to allow a fetus to pass from the uterus into the vagina and birthing canal; dilation is measured in centimeters.

DIRECT HEAT. Cooking food directly over a flame.

DOULA. Woman specially trained to support and assist women before, during, and after childbirth.

DUCTUS ARTERIOSUS. Fetal blood vessel connecting the pulmonary artery to the aorta, allowing oxygenated blood to bypass the fluid-filled lungs, and supply oxygen to the fetus.

E

EARLY LABOR. First phase of the first stage of labor, when contractions are regular but relatively mild.

EFFACEMENT. Thinning and shortening of the cervix, usually measured as a percentage to indicate the advancement of a pregnant woman's labor/delivery.

EFFLEURAGE. Massage maneuver performed with the whole hand or thumb, using long, gliding strokes.

ELECTRONIC FETAL HEART-RATE MONITOR (EFM). Device used during labor to monitor a baby's heart rate.

ENGAGEMENT. When the fetus is positioned within the pregnant woman's pelvis as a precursor to labor and delivery.

EPIDURAL ANESTHESIA. Pain medication given through a small catheter placed into a space around the spinal cord in the low back. It blocks pain in the lower half of the body.

EPISIOTOMY. Surgical incision of the woman's perineum (often performed pre-emptively to avoid tearing) to allow the fetus to more easily pass through the opening of the vagina.

ESTRIOL. Hormone measured as part of the Second Trimester Screening .

ESTROGEN. Hormone produced by females, levels of which increase during pregnancy; such increases can cause nausea, particularly during the first trimester.

F

FALSE LABOR. Signs of labor that occur before true labor begins: irregular contractions, etc.

FAMILIAL DYSAUTONOMIA (FD). Genetically inherited disease of the nervous system. Most common among Ashkenazi Jewish populations; cvs and amniocentesis can detect the disease prior to birth.

FAMILY PHYSICIAN. Medical doctor specializing in the primary care of patients of all ages, including both men and women.

FETAL MONITORING. Tracking fetal heart tones and expectant mother's contractions (usually with a high-tech medical electrode device) for indications of the baby's well-being during labor.

FETUS. Developing human in the womb.

FIRST STAGE OF LABOR. Stage of labor when a woman's body uses regular and escalating contractions to prepare for delivery.

FIRST TRIMESTER SCREENING (ALSO COMBINED SCREENING). Test for Down Syndrome, usually done between 10–14 weeks of pregnancy; includes ultrasound (to assess nuchal fold thickness), and two blood tests, for human chorionic gonadotropin (HCG) and pregnancy associated plasma protein A (PAPP-A).

FOLIC ACID. Nutrient that fosters red blood cell and hemoglobin formation, while also helping prevent neural tube defects in the fetus.

FALLOPIAN TUBES (OVIDUCTS). Fine tubes that lead from the ovaries to the uterus; where conception takes place.

FORCEPS. Tong-like instrument used to extract a fetus from the vagina.

FOREPLAY. Warm-up petting and other sexual behaviors performed prior to intercourse.

FRICTION. Massage maneuver using circular movements of thumbs and fingertips to penetrate and deeply work muscles.

FUNDUS. Upper section of the uterus.

GLUTEUS MUSCLES. Group of muscles comprising the buttocks; they make good targets for massage.

H

HOMO HABILIS. Ancestor of modern humans that lived two to three million years ago; believed to be the first to use tools, thus the name, which means "handy man" in Latin.

HOMO SAPIENS. Most advanced species of modern human (so far), "wise man" in Latin, and what the cultivated caveman should strive for.

HORMONES. Chemicals produced by glands in the body to help regulate bodily functions.

HUMAN CHORIONIC GONADOTROPIN (HCG). Hormone in women that prompts the ovaries to produce more estrogen and progesterone after conception.

HUMAN PLACENTAL LACTOGEN (HPL). Hormone produced by the placenta in pregnant women prompting a shift in metabolism to assist growth of the fetus. Also prepares breasts for milk production.

HYPNOSIS BIRTH. Act of laboring and/or giving birth while under self-hypnosis.

I

INDIRECT HEAT. Cooking food near but not directly over a flame.

INDUCTION DRUGS. Administered to begin or intensify uterine contractions during labor.

INHIBIN A. Hormone measured as part of the second trimester screening.

IRON. Nutrient crucial to production of blood.

J

JAUNDICE. Common condition in infants that gives a newborn's skin a yellowish tint, generally the result of an excess of bilirubin in the blood.

K

KAMA SUTRA. Sexual textbook written in India some 1,700 years ago by Vatsyayana.

KEGEL EXERCISES. Series of exercises pioneered by Dr. Arnold Kegel in the 1970s as a means of strengthening the pubococcygeus muscle to prepare a woman for labor. Kegel exercises are also used to treat urinary incontinence (leakage).

KNUCKLEDRAGGER. One whose knuckles scrape the ground when walking, a key identifying characteristic of a contemporary caveman.

L

LABOR. Process of birthing a child, usually divided into three stages

LABOR AND DELIVERY NURSE. Nurse with specialized training in labor and birth.

LACTATION. Production of milk in the female breasts.

LANUGO. Covering of soft hair sprouting from fetal hair follicles about five months into gestation; usually shed in the womb or soon after birth.

LIBIDO. Sexual desire or, as defined by Dr. Sigmund Freud, the energy supplied by one's primitive biological urges.

LISTERIOSIS. Rare food-borne bacterial illness that poses a risk to a developing fetus.

LOCHIA. Vaginal discharge that persists for a few days to a week or more after birth.

M

MASTITIS. Infection of the breast that afflicts some new mothers.

MECONIUM. Greenish-black, tar-like substance that typically comprises the baby's first bowel movement; unlike later feces, it is sterile and odorless.

MISSIONARY POSITION. Position for sexual intercourse, man on top, woman on the bottom, facing him.

MOLCAJETA. Central American version of the mortar and pestle, made from stone, often shaped like a pig.

MORNING SICKNESS. Nausea experienced by pregnant women; usually most intense in the morning, especially in the first trimester of pregnancy.

MORTAR. Bowl made of stone, ceramic or marble, companion to the pestle, used since prehistoric times as a vessel for holding smeared or crushed ingredients.

MUCUS PLUG. Cervical secretions that block the opening of the cervix during pregnancy.

N

NEANDERTHAL. Primitive species of human (Homo neanderthalensis) that lived during the Paleolithic period, some 30,000 to 230,000 years ago.

NEONATAL. State of being newborn.

NESTING INSTINCT. Urges and compulsions in expectant parents to complete tasks and prepare one's home for the arrival of a newborn.

NUCHAL TRANSLUCENCY. Ultrasound test to screen a fetus for the risk of Down Syndrome; usually done as part of first trimester screening between 10–14 weeks of pregnancy.

##

OB-GYN. Specialized physician who practices obstetrics (the care of a pregnant woman and fetus) and gynecology (care of the female reproduction system).

OVARY(IES). Twin organs that produce ova (eggs) in the female reproductive system.

OXYTOCIN. Hormone associated with labor in pregnant women; a synthetic form (pitocin) is often administered medically to induce, prolong, and intensify labor.

P

PAP SMEAR. Sampling of cervical cells examined to screen for abnormalities in the female reproductive system. Named for Dr. Georgios Papanikolaou (1883–1962), who invented the test.

PEDIATRICIAN. Specialized physician who cares for children.

PELVIC EXAM. Medical examination of the female reproductive system.

PERINEUM. External tissues surrounding the vagina, urethra, and anus; commonly refers to the tissue directly between the vagina and anus.

PESTLE. Miniature club or bat used since prehistoric times to grind and/or pulverize the contents of the mortar.

PETRISSAGE. Massage maneuver employing gentle grabbing and lifting of muscles away from the bone, followed by light rolling, pressing, and squeezing.

PICA. Rare, potentially dangerous disorder that drives pregnant women and young children to consume non-food substances such as soil, soap, paint, and paper.

PITOCIN. Artificial form of the hormone oxytocin, used to expedite labor.

PLACENTA. Blood-laden organ supplying oxygen and nourishment to a fetus.

PLACENTA PREVIA. Condition in pregnant women where the placenta covers part or all of the cervical opening in the uterus.

PLACENTAL ABRUPTION. Condition in which a pregnant woman's placenta prematurely separates from the uterine lining.

POSTPARTUM. After childbirth.

POSTPARTUM NURSE. Nurse who specializes in caring for mother and newborn after delivery.

PAPP-A. Pregnancy associated plasma protein-A measured as part of Second Trimester Screening.

PRE-ECLAMPSIA. Potentially dangerous (to the mother) disorder in pregnant women characterized by high blood pressure and protein in the urine; generally treated with prolonged bed rest.

PRENATAL. Prior to birth.

PRENATAL MASSAGE. Massage techniques designed specifically to benefit a pregnant woman.

PRENATAL MASSAGE THERAPIST. Massage expert who specializes in massage techniques benefiting pregnant women.

PRETERM LABOR. When the onset of labor begins sooner than 37 weeks of pregnancy.

PRIMIGRAVIDA. Woman experiencing pregnancy and childbirth for the first time.

PROGESTERONE. Hormone that promotes gestation through growth of uterine blood vessels; also essential for a normal menstrual cycle.

PROTEIN. Nutrient that serves as the main building block of fetal cell production.

PUBOCOCCYGEUS. Muscle at the base of the pubic region and the target of toning and strengthening through Kegel exercises.

PUMICE STONE. Volcanic rock with a coarse texture useful as an exfoliating tool for sloughing calluses and extra skin from the body.

R

RIPENING. Softening of the cervix allows for dilation and effacement.

S

SECOND STAGE OF LABOR. Period of time during labor when pushing begins (in a vaginal birth) and delivery occurs.

SECOND TRIMESTER SCREENING. Maternal blood test done between 15–20 weeks of pregnancy, measuring four substances: alpha-fetoprotein (AFP), human chorionic gonadotropin (HCG), estriol, and inhibin A. Provides risk assessment for Down Syndrome, Trisomy 18 and neural tube defects.

SICKLE CELL DISEASE. Genetically inherited group of disorders causing abnormal blood cells. Most common in the United States among African Americans, it is a chronic condition that varies in severity and may cause a combination of health problems including anemia, severe pain, and organ damage; cvs and amniocentesis can detect the disease prior to birth.

SPINAL BLOCK. Pain killing and pain masking drugs delivered via an injection to the lower spinal cord; often used during cesarean section surgery.

STATION. Location of a baby's head relative to certain points of the female pelvis, measured on a scale of 0 to +5; the high end of the scale is a baby's head at the crowning position at the opening of the vagina.

SUCKING REFLEX. Baby's instinct to search for the breast and mother's milk; known to linger later in life for many cavemen.

SURIBACHI AND SURIKOGI. Japanese version of the mortar and pestle, originated in southern China in the 11th century.

T

TAPOTEMENT. Massage maneuver involving a series of tapping motions applied with the edge of the hand, fingertips, or closed hand.

TAY-SACHS DISEASE (TSD). Genetically inherited fatal disorder of the brain and nervous system. Most common among Ashkenazi Jewish populations; cvs and amniocentesis can detect the disease prior to birth.

TERM. Full duration of a woman's pregnancy, typically 40 weeks from conception to delivery.

THIRD STAGE OF LABOR. After birth of the baby, when the woman delivers the placenta and amniotic sac.

TOCOLYTIC. Type of drug used to delay labor during pregnancy.

TOXOPLASMOSIS. Rare illness transmitted through contract with cat feces, uncooked meat, and other sources.

TRANSITION LABOR. Third and final phase of labor's first stage, in which contractions and labor-related symptoms are most acute.

TRIMESTER. One of three segments of the pregnancy term, lasting about three months.

u

ULTRASOUND (SONOGRAPHY). Medical technique using sound waves to create visual images of the interior of the human body.

UTERUS (WOMB). Pear-shaped muscular organ in a woman's pelvis that holds and nourishes a developing fetus.

v

VACUUM EXTRACTION. When traction is applied to the fetal head with a suction device to help with the delivery.

VAGINA. Muscular tube of the female anatomy leading to the cervix and uterus; the birth canal where a baby makes its way out during a vaginal birth.

VERNIX CASEOSA. Waxy, cheese-like substance that covers and protects the skin of the fetus, comprised mainly of oil and sloughed fetal skin cells.

VITAMIN A. Promotes healthy skin, eyesight, and bone and tooth growth in a fetus.

VITAMIN C. Promotes formation of healthy bones, teeth, and gums in a fetus, while helping expectant mom with iron absorption.

w

WATER BIRTH. Act of laboring and/or giving birth while partially submerged in water.

WHITE NOISE. Non-intrusive sound designed to mask other, more intrusive sounds, so as to soothe or encourage sleep.

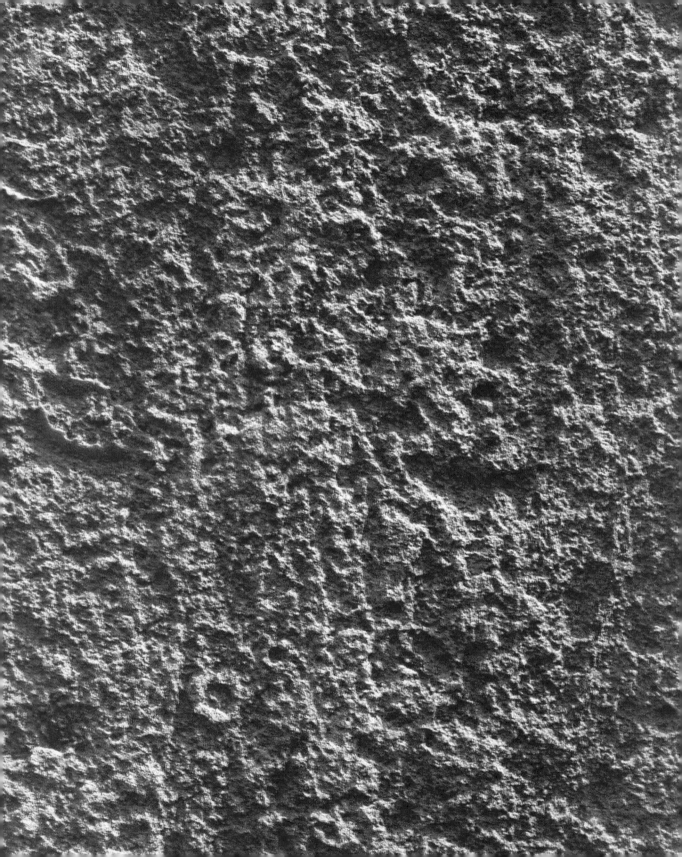

INDEX

A

Abortion, 76
  spontaneous, 79
Acetaminophen, 85
Aerobics, 109
Advil, 85
Afrin, 85
Afterbirth, 199, 211
Alcohol, 61, 75–76, 79, 82–83, 116
Aleve, 85
Allergy medication, 85
Alpha-fetoprotein (AFP), 71, 211
American Academy of Pediatrics (AAP),
  181
American Board of Obstetrics and
  Gynecology, 65
American College of Obstetricians and
  Gynecologists, 107, 181
Amniocentesis, 19, 72, 87, 211
Amniotic fluid, 72, 176, 188, 211
Amniotic sac, 68, 176, 211
Amniotomy, 188, 211
Androgens, 86
Anemia, 72
Anencephaly, 71
Antacids, 85
Anti-convulsants, 86
Antihistamines, 85
Anusol HC, 85
APGAR test, 201, 211
Asbestos, 30, 49
Asparagus Soup, 154–155
Aspirin, 85
Axid, 85

B

Babies
  beginning movements, 19
  developmental stages, 18, 19, 20
  due date caculations, 18
  fetal heartbeat, 18
  gestational diet for, 125
  indoor safety and, 48–49
  knowing sex of, 18
  music for, 39, 40
  names for, 20
  newborn appearance, 182
  opens eyes, 19
  organ development, 20
  outdoor safety and, 50
  reaction to light and sounds
    outside womb, 20
  secondhand smoke and, 39
  shifting in utero, 20
  size, trimester differences, 18, 19, 20
Bachelor friends, 38
Back pain, 22, 32, 74
Balance problems, 74
Basic Vinaigrette, 158
Baths
  for hemorrhoids, 74
  sexual activity and, 100
Bed rest, 83
Benadryl, 85
Benefiber, 85
Beverages, 166–169
  Cranberry Cooler, 168
  Gronk's Favorite Smoothie, 168
  Large Marge-arita, 167
  Manhattan, 167
  nutritious, 167, 168
  Piña Colada, 167
Biking, 109
Bilirubin, 201, 211
Birth announcements, 20
Birthing plan, 173, 211

Blood pressure, 20, 83
  age factor, 87
  exercise and, 111
  massage and, 42
  obesity and, 106
  placental abruption and, 82–83
  pregnancy-induced, 81
Breakfast, 135–139
Breakfast Strata, 137–138
Breastfeeding, 77, 200
Breast(s)
  colostrum production, 19
  disease, 86
  increased size, 19
  pump, 212
  tenderness, 18, 97
Breathing
  shortness of, 24
Budgets, 29–31
Butoconazole, 85

C

Caffeine, 75
Calcium, 63, 126–127, 212
Canavan disease, 72, 212
Cancer
  lung, 39
Carbohydrates, 127
Cardiopulmonary resuscitation (CPR),
  56–57, 212
Car safety, 50–51
  emergency kit, 50
  seats, 30, 50
Centers for Disease Control and
  Prevention (CDC)
  cesarean sections and, 196
  on obesity, 106
  on use of midwives, 65
Cephalopelvic disproportion (CPD),
  197, 212

Cervix, 68, 212
  dilation, 68, 185, 186, 187, 190,
    191, 193
  effacement, 185, 193, 213
  in first stage labor, 190
  flattening, 185, 186
  incompetent, 83
  ripening, 185, 218
Cesarean section, 83, 189, 196–197, 212
  age factor in, 87
  reasons for, 197
Changing tables, 52, 54, 55, 212
Childbirth
  assisted, 189, 211
  birthing plan, 173, 211
  breech, 67, 179, 189–190, 212
  by cesarean section, 83
  equipment, 180
  estimating date of, 62, 68
  fetal heart-rate monitor, 179
  at home, 67
  under hypnosis, 178, 215
  insurance for, 29
  labor and delivery, 171–207
  multiple, 67, 82, 197
  natural, 67, 76
  positions for, 195, 196
  premature, 83
  safety of, 64
  surviving rigors of, 12
  water birthing, 66, 178
Childcare
  planning for, 20
Chlorpheniramine, 85
Chorionic Villous Sampling (cvs), 72
Chromosomes, 71, 72
  abnormalities in, 72
Cimetidine, 85
Circumcision, 20, 77, 173, 212
Citrucel, 85
Claritin, 85
Classic American Lasagna Bolognese,
  150–151
Clitoris, 69
Clothing, baby, 29
  second-hand, 31
  yard sales, 31
Clotrimazole, 85
Coffee, 75, 135
Cold medications, 85
Colic, 202, 212
Colostrum, 19, 202, 212
Coltsfoot, 75

Comfrey, 75
Commission for the Accreditation of
  Birth Centers (cabc), 67
Communication, 92, 93, 94, 95
Conception, 212
Constipation, 20, 74, 85
Contractions, 212
  Braxton Hicks, 20, 175, 191, 212
  consistency in, 186
  duration of, 191
  in first stage labor, 191
  frequency, 191
  herbal remedies and, 86
  intensity, 191, 193
  magnitude, 193
  regular, 176, 190
  5-1-1 rule, 186
  strengthening, 188
Cooking, 113–169
  with alcohol, 116
  Asparagus Soup, 154–155
  bacon, 138
  Basic Vinaigrette, 158
  beverages, 166–169
  breakfast, 135–139
  Breakfast Strata, 137–138
  Classic American Lasagna Bolognese,
    150–151
  cleaning up from, 117
  compound butter, 144
  conversions in, 134
  Cranberry Cooler, 168
  cream cheese, 137
  doneness, 130
  eggs, 137, 138
  equipment, 133
  fish, 131
  following recipes, 131–132
  foods to avoid, 121
  on the grill, 140–148
  Grilled Pizza, 146–148
  Grilled Pork Tenderloin Salad,
    159–160
  Grilled Salsa, 164–165
  Gronk's Favorite Smoothie, 168
  Homemade Granola with Yogurt
    and Fresh Fruit, 139
  with hot peppers, 165
  Large Marge-arita, 167
  Lentil Soup, 153–154
  listeriosis and, 131
  Manhattan, 167
  Marinated Cucumber and Tomato
    Salad, 161
  measurements in, 134
  meats, 130
  one-pot, 148–155

  pasta, 149–151
  Pesto, 163–164
  Piña Colada, 167
  potatoes, 159
  rice, 152–153
  Risotto with Chicken, Artichoke,
    and Baby Spinach, 152–153
  with roux, 155
  safe food-handling, 117, 129
  salads, 156–161
  salsa, 160, 164–165
  sauces, 162–163
  shopping for, 122
  Shrimp and Vegetable Kebabs
    with Lemon, 145–146
  smoothies, 168
  soups, 153–155
  Southwest Flank Steak with
    Cilantro Butter, 143–144
  spice rubs, 143
  stocking pantry for, 119, 120
  strong odors and flavors, 121, 124
  tomato sauce, 151
  The World's Best Fluffy Pancakes,
    136
Couvade, 18, 22, 24, 32, 97, 213
Cradles, 52
Cranberry Cooler, 168
Cravings, food, 18, 123, 124
Cribs, 52, 54, 55
Cystic fibrosis, 72, 73, 213

D

Danazole, 86
Depression
  antepartum, 22
  clinical, 22, 32
  postpartum, 22, 24
Dextromethorphan, 85
Diabetes, 122
  age factor, 87
  exercise and, 111
  gestational, 67, 82
  obesity and, 106
  placental abruption and, 82–83
  preeclampsia and, 81
Diaper pails, 52
Diarrhea, 85
Diet, 8. See also Cooking
  balanced, 119, 122
  calcium in, 126
  carbohydrates in, 127
  fast food, 122

fats in, 127
folic acid, 127
health risks, 130, 131
hydration in, 124
iron, 63, 74, 125–126
junk food, 122, 123
nutritional needs, 125–128
pica and, 123, 125
processed foods, 122
protein in, 126–127
snacks, 122
vegetarian, 125
vitamins, 128
whole grains, 126
Dietary sources
calcium, 126
carbohydrates, 127
fat, 127
folic acid, 127
iron, 126
protein, 126–127
Digestion
massage and, 41
Diphenhydramine, 85
Doctors
appointments with, 18
choosing, 64
confirmation of pregnancy by, 18
family, 65, 214
obstetrician-gynecologist
(OB-GYN), 64–65
pediatricians, 19, 56
perinatologist, 65
referrals for, 64
regular visits, 20
training, 65
Doulas, 64, 66, 173, 213
Down syndrome
age factor, 87
testing, 71–72
Doxylamine, 85
Dristan, 85
Drugs, 61, 80
androgens, 86
anti-convulsant, 86
categories, 84, 86
danazole, 86
herbal, 84, 86
induction, 194, 215
lithium, 86
over-the-counter, 84, 85
pain relief, 66, 85
prescription, 84, 86
retinoids, 86
teratogenic, 86
tocolytic, 194
toxic, 86

Ductus arteriosus, 213
Due dates, 18

E

Eating disorders, 111
Echinacea, 86
Embryotoxicity, 80
Emotions
hormones and, 21, 22
Endometriosis, 86
Energy, 19
travel and, 28
Epidural anesthesia, 66, 173, 188–189,
194, 213
Episiotomy, 66, 173, 189, 196, 201, 214
Equipment, 2
budgeting for, 29–31
on the Internet, 30
nursery items, 52–53
second-hand, 30
trading pools for, 30–31
yard sales, 30
Escoffier, Auguste, 140
Estriol, 71, 214
Estrogen, 22, 23, 214
Exercise, 26, 106–112
aerobic, 109
cardiovascular, 108, 110–111, 212
cautions, 108–109, 110, 111
choices, 109
constipation and, 74
equipment, 109
hydration and, 112
joint, 18, 92, 107
Kegel, 19, 112, 215
monitoring body's behavior in, 109
personal trainer for, 108, 110
pilates, 109
pregnancy/delivery benefits of,
107, 110
prohibitions, 107
recommendations for, 107–108
safety issues, 76–77
snacks and, 112
strength training, 108, 111–112
stretching, 74, 108, 110
trouble signs, 112
yoga, 74, 108, 109

F

Fallopian tubes, 68–69, 214
Familial dysautonomia, 72, 214
Famotidine, 85
Fathers-to-be. See also Men as
pregnancy partners
changing bad/developing good
habits in anticipation, 37, 38
coping mechanisms for, 32
couvade symptoms, 18, 22, 24, 32
delivery room behavior, 195
diet, 8
in first stage labor, 192
in labor/delivery role, 171–207
mood variations in, 22
physical symptoms of stress, 32
projects/preparations for arrival,
35–56
protective instincts in, 19
responsibilities of, 16
in second stage labor, 198
sleep, 8, 16
smoking and, 38
stress and, 16, 22
in third stage labor, 199
Fatigue, 18, 22, 24, 74
muscle, 41
Fats, 127
Feet, swollen, 20
Femstat, 85
Fetal alcohol syndrome, 79
Feverfew, 86
Folic acid, 63, 127, 214
Food and Drug Administration (FDA), 84
Forceps, 180, 189, 214

G

Gardening, 51
Gas-X, 85
Gender identification, 72, 73
Genetic
counseling, 18
disorders/testing, 71–73
Ginkgo biloba, 86
Ginseng, 86
Goldenseal, 86
Golf, 109
Grilled Pizza, 146–148
Grilled Pork Tenderloin Salad, 159–160
Grilled Salsa, 164–165

Grilling, 140–148
  equipment, 141–142
  Grilled Pizza, 146–148
  Shrimp and Vegetable Kebabs
    with Lemon, 145–146
  Southwest Flank Steak with
    Cilantro Butter, 143–144
Gronk's Favorite Smoothie, 168
Guaifenesin, 85
Gyne-Lotrimin, 85

H

Headaches, 74, 86
Health and medical issues
  abortion, 76
  for African Americans, 72
  alcohol, 61, 75–76, 79, 82–83
  for Ashkenazi Jews, 72
  asymptomatic bacteriuria, 81
  caffeine, 75
  for Caucasian/Northern Europeans,
    73
  circumcision, 20, 77–78
  constipation, 74
  drugs, 61, 80
  environmental toxins, 79–81
  genetic testing, 71–73
  gestational diabetes, 67
  group B streptococci, 81
  harmful vapors, 79–80
  hemorrhoids, 74
  herpes, 80
  HIV, 80
  jaundice, 82
  lead exposure, 80
  neurological, 79
  nutrients, 62, 63
  organic solvents, 79–80
  placental abruption, 82–83
  placenta previa, 83
  preeclampsia, 67, 81
  prenatal care, 69–86
  prenatal vitamins, 62–63
  preterm labor, 82
  sexually transmitted diseases, 80
  smoking, 38, 39, 76, 79, 82
  teratogens, 79–81
  toxoplasmosis, 80
  travel, 75
  urinary tract infection, 81
Heartburn, 41, 74, 85
Hemorrhoids, 74, 85
Herbal tea, 75

Herpes
  genital, 197
  simplex, 80
Hiking, 109
Hippocrates, 116
HIV, 80
Hobbies, 26
Homemade Granola with Yogurt
  and Fresh Fruit, 139
Home projects/preparations, 18, 35–56
  additions, 30
  hazards, 30
  nursery, 20
  safety issues, 48–51
Hormones, 18, 23–24, 215
  androgen, 86
  balance in, 19
  cravings and, 124
  emotions and, 21, 22
  estrogen, 22, 23, 214
  functions of, 23, 24
  human chorionic gonadotropin, 23
  human placental lactogen, 23
  insulin, 82
  massage and, 41
  oxytocin, 23, 191
  placental, 82
  progesterone, 24, 218
  regulation of pregnancy functions
    by, 23
  relaxin, 110
  testosterone, 23
Hospital/birthing center, 65–67
  birthing suites in, 66
  choice of healthcare providers
    and, 64
  home, 67
  maternity wards, 183–185, 201
  packing for, 20
  planning route to, 20
  postpartum stay, 202, 203
  preparing for, 173–176
  preregistration at, 20
  rooming-in options in, 66
  touring, 19
  water-birthing capabilities in,
    66, 179
Hot tubs, 75
Human chorionic gonadotropin (HCG),
  23, 71, 215
Human placental lactogen, 23, 215
Hydrocortisone, 85
Hyperthermia, 80
Hypnosis, 178, 215
Hypoxia, 80

I

Ibuprofen, 85
Imodium, 85
Infections
  asymptomatic bacteriuria, 81
  group B streptococci, 81–82
  herpes, 80
  HIV, 80
  resistance to, 71
  respiratory, 39
  sexually transmitted, 80
  toxoplasmosis, 51, 80, 129–130
  urinary tract, 77, 81
Inhibin A, 71, 215
Insulin, 82
Insurance
  automobile, 50
  government, 55–56
  health, 18, 29, 55
  healthcare providers and, 64
  precertification for birthing facility,
    29
Internet
  baby equipment on, 30
  birthcenter website, 67
  marrow donor websites, 78
  umbilical cord blood websites, 78
Intimacy
  maintaining, 40
Iron, 63, 74, 125–126, 215

J

Jaundice, 82, 201, 215
Jogging, 109

K

Kama Sutra, 96, 101, 215
Kava kava, 86
Kegel exercises, 19

L

Labia minora/majora, 69
Labor, 171–207
  active, 193, 211
  amniotomy in, 188
  average length, 178
  birthing plan, 173, 211
  cervix during, 68 (See also Cervix)

complications and, 173
drugs during, 194
early, 213
encouraging, 23
epidural in, 188–189
expediting, 175
false, 175, 186–188, 214
fetal heart-rate monitor, 179
first stage, 176–178, 184, 190–193, 214
inducing, 176, 187
massage during, 41
observers, 180
preterm, 70, 75, 82, 83, 103, 217
second stage, 184, 193–198, 218
stages of, 184
third stage, 184, 199
transition, 193, 195
true, 186–188
Lactation, 202, 215
Lactic acid, 41
Lanugo, 216
Large Marge-arita, 167
Lead exposure, 80
Lentil Soup, 153–154
Listeriosis, 131, 216
Lithium, 86
Lobelia, 75
Lochia, 201, 216
Loperamide, 85
Loratadine, 85

M

Maalox, 85
Manhattan, 167
Marinated Cucumber and Tomato
    Salad, 161
Massage
    for father-to-be, 34
    prenatal, 19, 27, 40–48, 100, 217
Massage, prenatal, 217
    circulation and, 41
    contraindications for, 41–42
    digestion and, 41
    effleurage, 44, 213
    focus of, 42–43
    friction, 44
    hormone levels and, 41
    during labor, 41
    oils for, 43
    pain relief from, 41
    petrissage, 44, 217
    positioning for, 45–47

preparation for, 42
professional, 48
as seduction tool, 41
settings for, 42
sexual activity and, 100
sleep and, 41
stress relief and, 41
stretch marks and, 41
Swedish, 44
tapotement, 44, 218
techniques, 43–47
tools for, 42
vibration in, 44
Mastitis, 202, 216
Meals. See Cooking; Diet
Meconium, 202, 216
Men as pregnancy partners
    activities for couples, 33–34
    benefits of, 8–9
    communication and, 92, 93, 94, 95
    cooking and, 19, 20, 113–169
    couples relationship and, 89–112
    in labor/delivery role, 171–207
    massage, 19
    medical issues, 59–87
    projects/preparations for arrival
        for, 35–56
    rites of passage for, 16
    sacrifices expected, 16
    single-sex activities for, 33–34
Menstrual periods
    estimating delivery date and, 62, 68
Mental retardation, 71, 79, 80
Metamucil, 85
Miconazole, 85
Midwives, 64, 65, 173
Milk thistle, 86
Miscarriage, 18, 19, 83
    invasive testing and, 72
    sexual activity and, 103
Monistat, 85
Moods
    variable, 18, 21, 22
Morning sickness. See Nausea
Mothers-to-be
    age factor, 87
    anatomy of, 67–69
    aversions, 19, 124
    back pain, 74
    breast tenderness, 18
    clothing for, 19
    constipation, 74
    fatigue and, 18, 22, 74
    feels movement, 19

frequent urination, 18, 19, 20, 74
heartburn, 74
hemorrhoids, 74
hormonal activity
nausea, 1, 14, 18, 22, 74
nutritional needs, 118, 119
shortness of breath, 74
sleep and, 74
snacking, 20
varicose veins, 74
weight gain, 19
Motrin, 85
Music, 39, 40, 42
Mylanta, 85

N

Names, 20, 92
Naproxen, 85
Nausea, 1, 14, 18, 22, 74, 97, 100, 121,
    193, 216
Nesting instinct, 18, 92, 104, 216
Neural tube defects, 71, 72
Nizatidine, 85
Nuchal translucency, 71, 214, 216
Nursery
    carpeting in, 54
    colors in, 54
    equipment for, 30, 54, 55
    preparation, 53–55
    sleep and, 54
    window coverings, 55
Nurses, 64, 182–183
    anesthetist, 188
    importance of, 182–183
    labor and delivery, 182–183, 201, 215
    midwife, 65
    postpartum, 183, 201, 217
    rapport with, 182
    responsibilities of, 183
    training, 65

O

Obesity, 106, 122
Obstetrician-gynecologists, 6, 64
Ovaries, 19, 24, 68, 216
Ovulation, 24
Oxytocin, 23, 191, 194, 217

P

Paint, lead, 49
Parental care
  examples in nature, 6–7
Parenting/birthing classes, 19, 20, 92, 104–105
Pennyroyal, 75
Perinatologists, 65
Perineum, 69
Pesto, 163–164
Pets, 20, 50–51
Phenylketonuria, 111
Pica, 123, 125
Pilates, 108
Piña Colada, 167
Pitocin, 23, 187, 217
Placenta, 24, 68, 69, 78, 217
  delivery of, 184
  function of, 69
Placental abruption, 82–83, 217
  cesarean section and, 197
Placenta previa, 75, 83, 217
  age factor, 87
  cesarean section and, 197
  sexual activity and, 103
Preeclampsia, 67, 81, 217
  exercise and, 111
Pregnancy
  ambivalent feelings in, 12, 13
  anatomy and, 67–69
  back pain, 22
  body image issues in, 22
  conception and, 61, 62
  developments during, 15–34
  discomforts in, 20
  gestational milestones, 17–20
  "glow," 19
  high-risk, 64
  insecurity over, 12, 13
  intimacy during, 92
  medical aspects, 59–87
  medications during, 84–86
  milestones in, 14
  nausea in, 22
  physical symptoms, 22
  prenatal care and, 69–86
  "sympathetic," 24
  tests, 18, 61, 62
  timing high and low points of, 14
Pregnancy associated plasma protein-A (PAPP-A), 71
Prenatal care, 69–86
  laboratory tests, 70

Pap smear, 70
pelvic exam, 70
physical exams, 69, 70
radiology tests, 70
Primigravida, 14, 217
Progesterone, 24, 218
Protein, 126–127, 218
Pseudoephedrine, 85
Pseudofed, 85
Pubococcygeus, 218

R

Radon, 30, 49
Ranitidine, 85
Reproductive organs, 68, 69
Retinoids, 86
Risotto with Chicken, Artichoke, and Baby Spinach, 152–153
Robitussin, 85
Rocking chairs, 55

S

Safety issues, 48–51, 80
  car, 50
  cardiopulmonary resuscitation (CPR), 56–57
  in cooking, 117
  exercise, 76–77
  fire escape route, 56
  first aid kit, 56
  indoor, 48–49
  outdoor, 50
  pets, 50–51
St. John's wort, 86
Salads, 156–161
  Basic Vinaigrette, 158
  dressings, 156–158
  Grilled Pork Tenderloin Salad, 159–160
  ingredients, 157
  Marinated Cucumber and Tomato Salad, 161
Sassafras, 75
Sauces, 162–163
Sciatica, 74
Seizures, 111
Sexual activity, 92, 96–103
  changing body proportions and, 99–100
  decline in, 18, 97

discomfort and, 99
effect on baby, 99
hormonal factors, 99
increase in, 19
"jumpstart labor," 20, 98, 100, 176
lack of desire for, 98, 99
lack of energy for, 19
massage and, 100
mental factors in, 97
miscarriage and, 103
obstacles to, 75
physical factors in, 97
positions, 101–103
during pregnancy, 73, 75
prohibitions against, 83, 103
snuggling, 101
Shower, baby, 30
Shrimp and Vegetable Kebabs with Lemon, 145–146
Sickle cell anemia, 72, 218
Simethicone, 85
Skin
  infections, 81–82
  irritations, 42
  stretch marks, 41
Sleep, 8, 16, 206
  and choosing room for nursery, 54
  insomnia, 74
  interruptions, 22
  massage and, 41
Smoking, 38, 76, 79
  preterm labor and, 82
  secondhand smoke and, 39, 79
  SIDS and, 79
Social security, 204
Southwest Flank Steak with Cilantro Butter, 143–144
Spina bifida, 71
Sports, 109
Stress, 32
  behavioral manifestations of, 22
  massage and, 41
  on pets, 50
  relieving, 25–28, 91
  sources of, 16
Stretch marks, 41, 78
Strollers, 52
Sucking reflex, 202, 218
Supplements
  dietary, 213
  iron, 126
Swimming, 109, 110
Syphilis, 80

T

Tagamet, 85

Tay-Sachs disease, 72, 219

Teratogens, 79–81

Testing
    alpha-fetoprotein, 71
    amniocentesis, 72
    anencephaly, 71
    blood, 70, 71
    Canavan disease, 72
    Chorionic Villous Sampling, 72
    cystic fibrosis, 72, 73
    Down Syndrome, 71–72
    estriol, 71
    familial dysautonomia, 72
    genetic, 71–73
    glucose screening, 82
    human chorionic gonadotropin, 71
    inhibin A, 71
    invasive, 72
    laboratory, 70
    miscarriage and, 72
    neural tube defects, 71, 72
    non-invasive, 71–72
    nuchal translucency, 71
    Pap smear, 70
    pregnancy, 18, 19, 61, 62
    radiology, 70
    sequential, 71
    sickle cell anemia, 72
    spina bifida, 71
    Tay-Sachs disease, 72, 219
    urinalysis, 70

Testosterone, 23

Toxoplasmosis, 51, 80, 129–130

Travel, 92
    by air, 75
    restrictions, 27–28

Trimester, first
    characteristics of, 18
    genetic testing, 71
    sexual activity in, 100

Trimester, second
    characteristics of, 19
    genetic testing, 71–72
    preeclampsia and, 81
    sexual activity in, 100
    travel during, 92

Trimester, third
    characteristics of, 20
    preeclampsia and, 81
    sexual activity in, 100

Trisomy 18, 71

Trisomy 21, 71–72

Tucks Pads, 85

Tums, 85

Tylenol, 85

U

Ultrasound, 66, 69, 70, 219
    pregnancy dating and, 70
    sex of baby and, 19

Umbilical cord, 69
    blood from, 78
    prolapse, 197, 213

Uterus, 68, 176, 190, 219
    blood vessel growth, 24
    placenta in, 69
    ruptured, 197

Utrasound
    genetic testing and, 71

V

Vacuum extraction device, 189

Vagina, 69, 219
    bleeding, 103
    yeast infection, 85

Valeria, 86

Varicose veins, 42, 74, 78, 110–111

Vernix caseosa, 19, 219

Vitamins, 128, 219
    deficiencies, 80
    diet and, 124
    prenatal, 62–63, 121, 128

Vulva, 69

W

Walking, 109

Water breaking, 20, 176, 188

Weight, baby's, 18, 19, 17620
    increases in, 20
    low, 79, 202

Weight, mother's
    gain, 19, 76

White noise, 54, 219

Womb. See Uterus

The World's Best Fluffy Pancakes, 136

Y

Yeast infection, 85

Yoga, 74, 108

Z

Zantac, 85

CAVE NOTES

CAVE NOTES

CAVE NOTES

CAVE NOTES

CAVE NOTES

ACKNOWLEDGMENTS

Transforming two contemporary Cro-Magnon types into published authors wouldn't have been possible without the efforts and contributions of a great many people. Special thanks to members of the Caveman's Ad Hoc Female Advisory Council (Colorado Chapter): **Kelli Jennings**, a registered dietician and prenatal nutritional expert who founded Apex Nutrition in Crested Butte (check out www.apexnutritionllc.com); **Desirae Mannering**, founder and director of Pregnancy, Birth & Beyond in Denver, a registered doula and certified prenatal massage therapist (visit www.pregnantbirth.com for more info); and **Missy Griffin**, a registered nurse specializing in labor and delivery who also serves as coordinator of the parent education department at Rose Medical Center in Denver (www.rosebabies.com).

We also owe a huge debt of gratitude to the numerous other council members who provided inspiration, support, constructive criticism, and admonishment throughout the writing of this book: **Emily Port**, **Jane Port**, **Candace Port-Hull**, and **Jennifer Port**; and **Bridget Ralston**, **Diana Ralston**, and **Juliette Ralston**. Our wives Emily and Diana deserve special commendation (and a lifetime of on-demand foot massages) for having the patience and fortitude to endure pregnancy and to keep an eye on the kids when we were holed up to write. Also, big unibrowed butterfly kisses to our newest cavelings, **Lila Port** and **Zane Ralston**, each of whom arrived during the writing.

We're especially grateful to **Susan Ralston** for her sage advice during our initial efforts to get a book published, and to **George Scott** of Scott & Nix for his patient, incisive, and always affable guidance on every aspect of this project. This book would not have been possible without his strong grasp of the caveman mindset (it takes one to know one) and the nurturing he offered his caveman authors. Cave-kudos go out to **Charles Nix** for creating a handsome and thoughtful design, and to **Gideon Kendall** for all the appropriately hilarious illustrations. We're also deeply indebted to **Nathaniel Marunas**, **Ruth O'Brien**, and **Bruce Lubin**, and the publishing team at Sterling for letting us unleash Gronk on the literary world.

We're indebted to **Brian Ralston**, M.D., F.A.A.F.P., for his vast—and always humorous—contributions to the book, and to **Paul Port** for the Gronk visage and for other bizarrely creative inspirations. We also wish to acknowledge Dr. Brian's colleague, **Charles J. Adamczyk**, M.D., F.A.A.F.P., whose insightful recommendations were invaluable to the medical sections.

Muchas gracias to the smiling folks at Diedrich's Garage Coffee Shop for the positive, caffeine-fueled karma, and to the fine people at RP Publishing for their support over the years. Thanks as well to the dedicated and professional folks at Gunnison Valley Hospital. And finally, thanks to **Charles Darwin** for postulating that we human beings can indeed evolve.

—DAVE PORT AND JOHN RALSTON
March, 2006

CAVE NOTES